I0415576

TABLE OF CONTENTS

INTRODUCTION

Human health and the practice of medicine are being revolution-ized by rapidly accelerating innovations. The innovations are ex-citing, in some cases life changing. And, they are coming from many disciplines including robotics, artificial intelligence, big data, supercomputing, augmented and virtual reality, genetics, bioengineering, materials science and much more.

Some examples of the latest medical innovations that we show-case:

- Cardiologists using augmented reality for 3D precision during heart surgery
- Digital glasses that restore sight
- Your brain staying young and learning for a lifetime
- Ending malaria by gene mutation
- Gene editing as a successful treatment for Muscular Dystrophy
- First example of Bioelectric medicine: tiny, biodegrad-able, wireless implants
- Robot healthcare givers
- Implants powered by the heart's kinetic energy
- Whole body regeneration
- Lab on a chip that detects cancer much faster
- eBandages that accelerate healing
- Smart patches monitoring your heart and health
- Ingestible electronic pills, controlled by your smart-phone with precision drug delivery

These are just a few examples of the remarkable medical cures and breakthroughs that we cover in the book. As a national jour-nalist, I've written the innovation developments as crisp, professional news summaries. They serve as a handy guide and provide you with the key facts you need to know.

I hope you enjoy exploring these fascinating medical break-throughs as much as I enjoyed researching and reporting them.

Thanks and best,

Ed Kane, Author of the 8 book series "Important Innovations Collection"

AUTHOR'S BIOGRAPHY

Ed Kane is the author of eight books on innovation. He created and serves as Executive Producer of CEO Global Foresight. CGF is a national program on PBS focused on breakthrough innovation changing our lives for the better. Guests have included the CEO's of Bayer AG, DARPA (the US Defense Department's Advanced Research Projects Agency), Terrafugia which created the world's first flying car and Adidas AG.

He also created and served as Executive Producer of CEO Corner originally for Bloomberg Radio. It was an hour interview program with the world's most innovative and entrepreneurial CEO's. Ed moved the program to television. It has aired on New England Cable News (NECN) for fifteen years. Guests have included the CEO's of Comcast, P&G, ExxonMobil and Verizon.

Ed is a science graduate of the University of Pennsylvania. He is an avid researcher into the future of breakthrough innovation and its impact on humanity.

1. **Your Brain, Lifetime Learning: Continuous Supply of New Neurons**

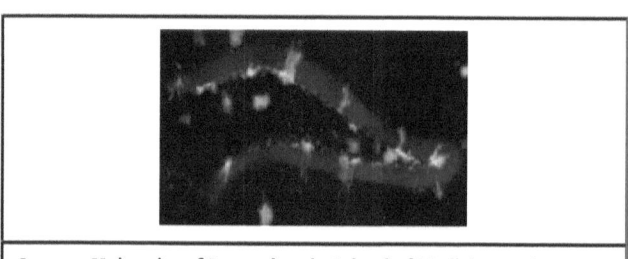

Source: University of Pennsylvania School of Medicine Brain Image

Important Discovery by University of Pennsylvania Medical School Scientists

This is breakthrough research from the University of Pennsylvania School of Medicine. The scientists have shown for the first time that brain neurons grow and develop over a lifetime from a single population of stem cells in the hippocampus region of the brain. That region is the brain's center of memory and learning. It's also a key area of reaction to stress and mood adjustments.

Why is This Important to You

The discovery underscores how a continuous supply of new neurons throughout life is the source of youthful like learning and memory throughout your life. The discovery was found in research on mice. And, it sets a new benchmark. It helps neuroscientists to determine how to enable youthful life brain conditions for memory and learning for all of us throughout our lives. It's also a path of discovery to repair and regenerate parts of the brain damaged by injury and aging. It's important new innovation and discovery enabled by neuroscientists at The University of Pennsylvania - my Alma mater.

2. **Implants Powered by a Beating Heart: New Device Captures Heart Energy**

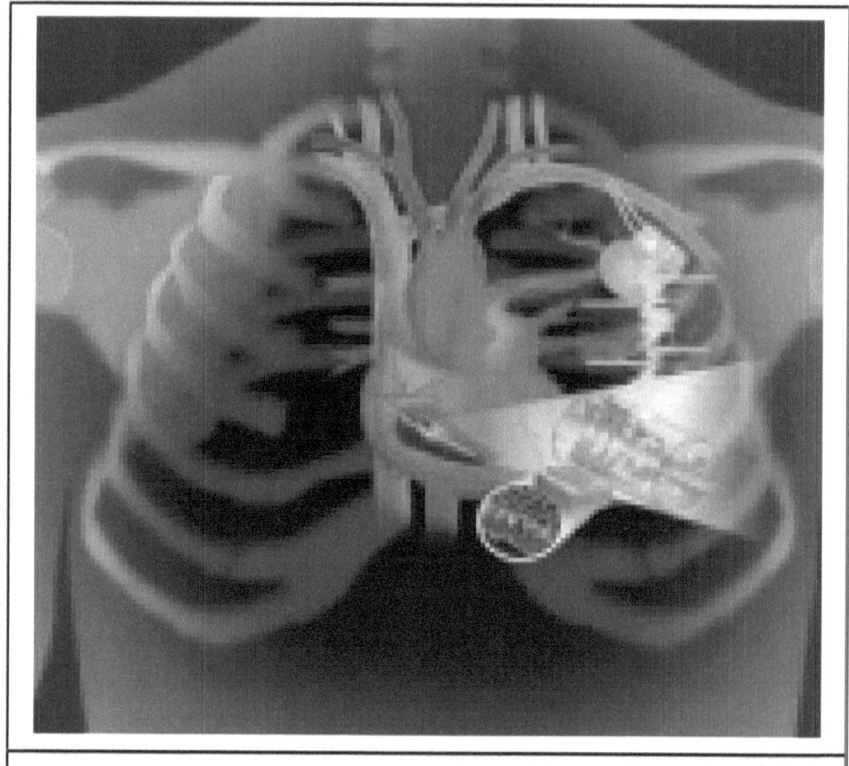

Source: Dartmouth College

Implants Powered By Electricity from Heart Beats

This is fascinating and very promising research from Dartmouth College engineers funded by the National Institute of Health (NIH), The Dartmouth team have created a dime sized device that harvests the kinetic energy of a beating heart to generate electricity and power a biomedical device indefinitely. It's an implant, a heart pacemaker, powered by a beating heart.

Dime-Sized Device

What is so interesting is this is a dime sized device. It relies on a thin film - piezoelectric film - attached to a pacemaker's lead. It converts heart beats' kinetic energy into electricity to power the pacemaker implant.

NIH Funded Research with Other Implant Device Applications

This is essentially an organ energy harvesting device that could work beyond the heart and for other organs such as kidneys. The Dartmouth team's three years of research results have been published in Advanced Materials Tech. They have two more years of NIH funding to complete testing and regulatory approval. A commercial product is expected in five years. It's a case of recapturing the heart's motion to give a new lease on life.

3. Cardiologists Using AR for Heart Surgery: 3D Precision

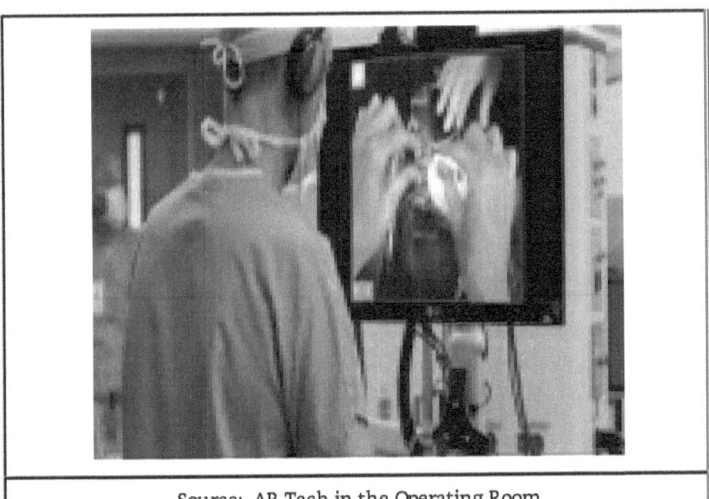

Source: AR Tech in the Operating Room

AR Goggles in the OR
Augmented reality is a technology that superimposes computer generated information on the user's view of the real world. It's being tested at Beth Israel Deaconess Medical Center in Boston. And it seems to greatly help surgeons visualize complex medical data particularly during heart surgery.

Surgeons with AR Goggles
A new self-contained AR device provides surgeons with the opportunity to interactively explore data in 3D and real time during complex surgical procedures. Here's how it works. The sur-

geon wears AR goggles that are similar to the glass screens worn by divers. The AR images are projected onto the surgeon's facial screen to augment their view and provide vital information on their patient during complex surgical procedures.

NIH Funded Successful Test Pilot Program

This is a pilot program and has been used successfully on 5 animal models. The program is supported by the National Institute of Health and is being expanded. The doctors and researchers say the technology so far has exciting potential. It allows doctors to superimpose images like MRI and CT scans as a guide during the operation. They say it helps guide treatment and patient care, eventually for humans.

4. Time Travelling Neuroscience: Caltech Research Breakthrough

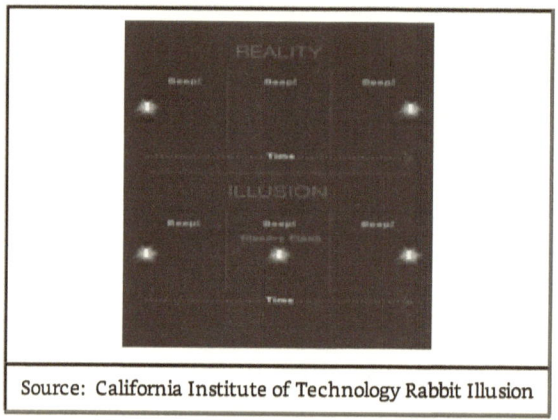

Source: California Institute of Technology Rabbit Illusion

How the Brain Retroactively Computes Rapid Audio & Visual Stimuli

Researchers at California Institute of Technology have developed two new illusions to document time travelling. The illusions, called The Rabbit Illusions as tracked above, reveal how the senses influence each other as they are received at rapid speed by the brain. In particular, how sound can trigger and create visual illusions after the fact.

Time Travel through "Postdiction" by the Brain

With the onrush of sensory perceptions to the brain, the illusions occur so rapidly that they trigger a brain phenomenon called postdiction as opposed to prediction. Postdiction happens when a stimulus that occurs later can retroactively affect our perception of an earlier event. That's time-traveling at the pure scientific research level.

Innovative and Breakthrough Neuroscience

The Caltech research is the first to show this type of time travelling illusion in the brain across multiple senses. It demonstrates how stimuli detected later can affect the brain's perception of stimuli that already occurred. The ground breaking research has been published in the journal PLOS One.

5. Bioelectric Medicine First: Biodegradable, Wireless, Tiny Implants

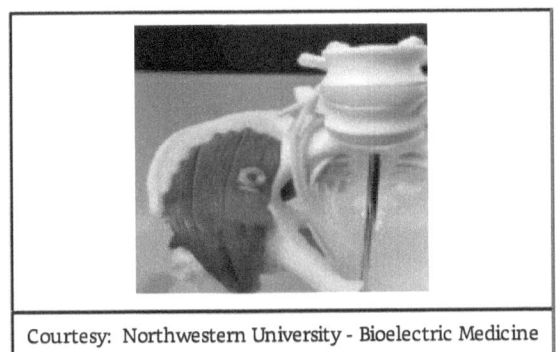

Courtesy: Northwestern University - Bioelectric Medicine

Pulses of Electricity to Accelerate Nerve Regeneration

Northwestern University researchers and Washington University neurosurgeons have developed the first example of bioelectric medicine. It's an implantable, biodegradable, wireless device. It speeds nerve regeneration and improves healing by pulses of electricity targeted directly at the site.

Size of a Dime

The implant is tiny. It's the size of a dime and has the thickness of a piece of paper. It delivers pulses of electricity to damaged nerves. In lab tests on post-operative animals, it proved very successful in accelerating the regeneration of nerves and enhancing the recovery of muscle strength and control.

Naturally Disappears

In a week or two, the implant biodegrades, is naturally absorbed into the body and totally disappears. The next steps will be testing it on humans. The research team believes that such temporary, short term, engineered devices, applied directly to the problem site, can complement or replace regular pharma treatment for a variety of medical conditions. This breakthrough innovation was published in the journal Nature Medicine.

6. Israeli Vision: Very High Tech, Digital Eyewear

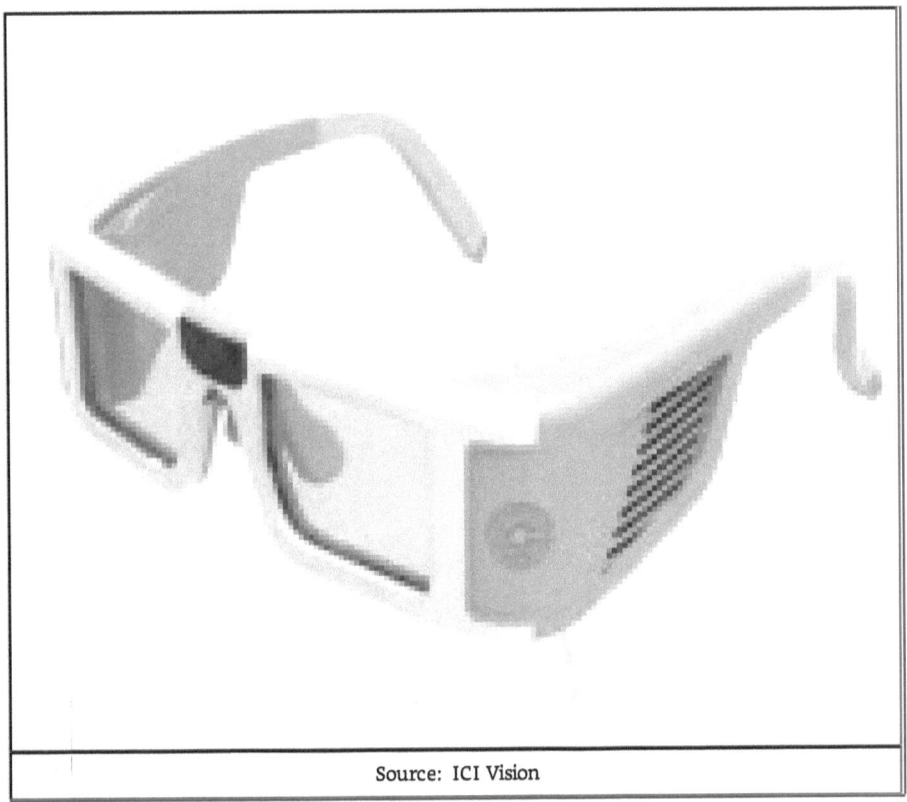

Source: ICI Vision

Israel's ICI Vision

ICI Vision of Tel Avis has developed very high tech eyewear for those with vision disabilities. Their Enhanced Vision Engine (EVE) is a fusion of hardware and software systems that combine AI, computer vision, mini HD cameras and proprietary eye tracking algorithms to bring sight to the virtually blind.

Digital Eyewear Platform with AI and HD Cameras

The technology in the glasses fills in the gaps in the individual's eyesight and projects images to healthy areas of the retina. The company calls it the first of its kind, individually optimized digital eyewear platform. The glasses are designed to help the visually impaired better navigate and help to correct blind spots.

7. Whole Body Regeneration – Genetic Switches: Harvard

Research

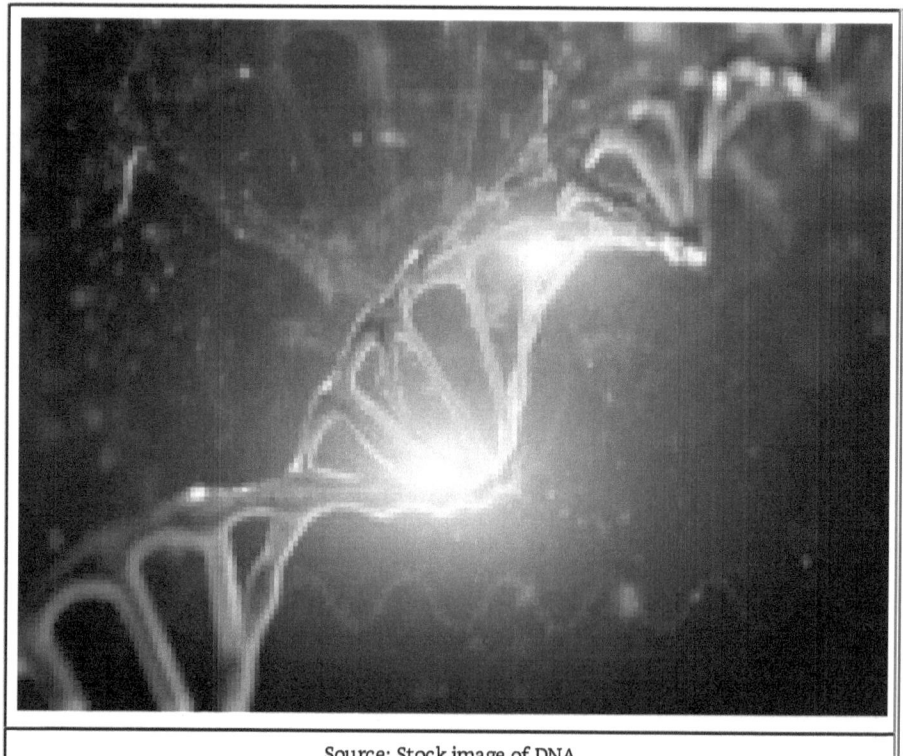

Source: Stock image of DNA

Salamanders, Geicos, Worms DNA

Harvard scientists started with a simple question: if some animals can regenerate parts of their bodies and even whole-body
regeneration, why can't I? The findings from their innovative
research are astounding. They've uncovered a number of DNA
switches that appear to control genes used in whole body regeneration. Their research is documented in the journal Science.

3 Banded Panther Worms

Examples of body regeneration, such as restoration of a severed
leg or tail, in the animal kingdom include salamanders, geicos
and worms. The team used 3 banded panther worms that can regenerate. Their findings: a section of non-coding DNA controls
the activation of a "master control gene" called early growth response or EGR. The EGR controls a number of other processes by

switching genes on and off.

Tip of the Iceberg
The team says their findings are just the tip of the iceberg of what accounts for regeneration in some animals. But they are the first to document that it starts with a master control gene switching other genes on and off.

8. Microneedle Patch Kills Infection and Delivers Safer Vaccines

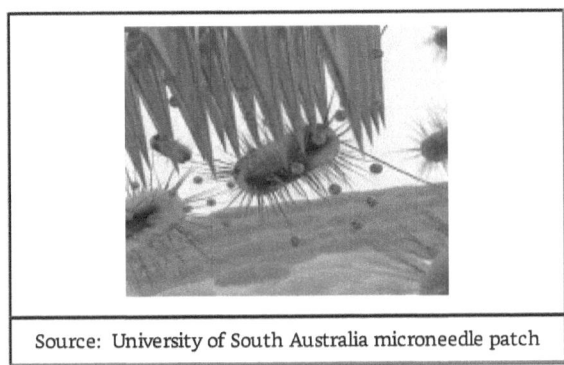

Source: University of South Australia microneedle patch

Silver Nanoparticles Kill Bacteria
Scientists at the University of South Australia have developed a microneedle patch embedded with silver nanoparticles and vaccine. It offers an alternative to traditional needle injections and eliminates infections at the injection site.

Alternative to Traditional Needles
The patch carries an array of microneedles that contain both vaccine and silver nanoparticles. When attached to the skin, the microneedles dissolve in one minute. The patch is painless, doesn't need to be refrigerated and releases the vaccine into the top layer of skin, not reaching any nerves. The vaccine is released into the bloodstream and the silver nanoparticles kill any bacteria. Bottom-line: it enables safer vaccinations and prevents infections. The team believes it would be particularly effective in

the developing world where vaccinations with unsterile needles result in infections.

9. New Lab on a Chip: Detects Cancer Faster

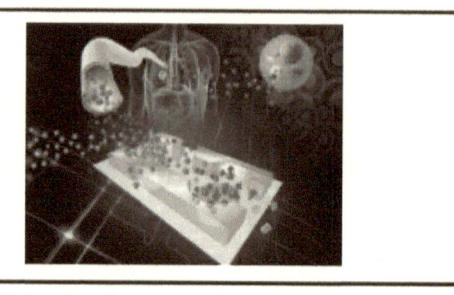

Source: University of Kansas Medical Center Lab on a Chip

Works On a Miniscule Amount of Plasma

The new, lab on a chip's key piece of innovation is a 3D nano-engineering method that mixes and senses biological elements based on a herringbone structure found in nature. The herringbone drains the liquid sample into a gap allowing hard contact with the surface of the chip system to recognize disease quickly. This is another example of nature inspired innovation.

Ultrasensitive Medical Device

This is an ultrasensitive diagnostic device developed at the University of Kansas Medical School. It's designed to enable doctors to detect cancer much faster from a drop of blood or plasma. That means earlier intervention and potentially better outcomes for patients. It's been successfully tested using clinical samples from ovarian cancer patients.

10. Inspiring AI Innovator: New AI that Predicts Pandemics

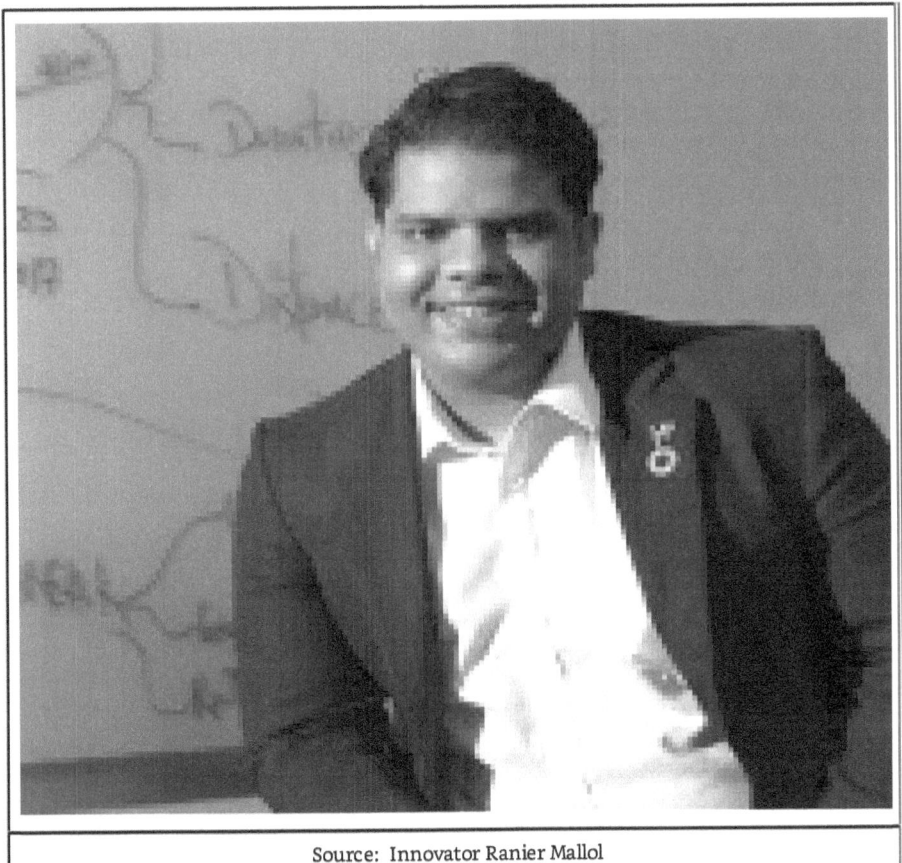

Source: Innovator Ranier Mallol

Inspiring Innovator - Young Scientist from the Dominican Republic

This new, AI predictive system is breakthrough and the innovator behind it is inspirational. Scientist Ranier Mallol of the Dominican Republic almost lost his mother to dengue fever when he was a boy. He vowed to do something about the disease, carried by mosquitos, which infects 390 million people every year. He developed an AI algorithm that is a breakthrough.

Aime

Mallol fed the algorithm that he developed statistics on dengue infections. The algorithm uses health, location, climate and socio-economic data to predict disease outbreaks three months before they happen. Its success rate is 88% accuracy. Mallol has established an organization called Aime that uses his algorithm to forecast disease outbreaks.

Predicts Dengue Plus

Mallol says his system is nationally implemented in Malaysia. And its uses are many including for Zika. And he is now developing it for diabetes.

11. Personalized Vitamins: Customized to the Individual

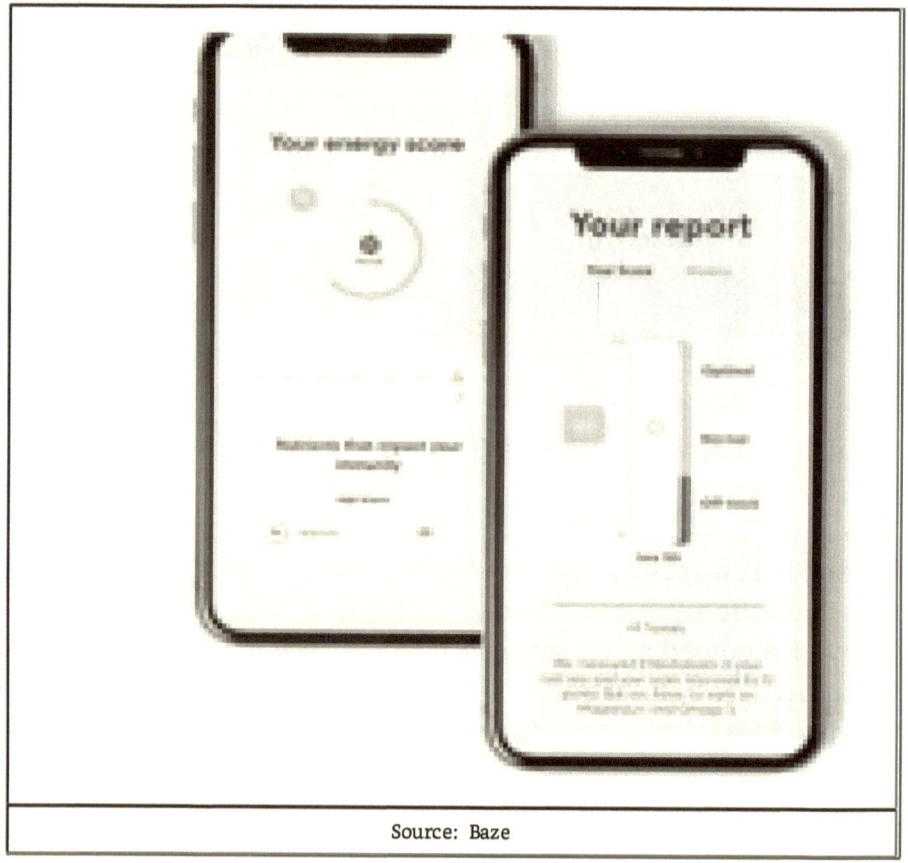

Source: Baze

Baze - Optimal, Personalized Dose Approach

Baze calls it the only evidence-based personalized vitamin service. The company has created a personalized vitamin system that provides optimal doses of vitamin nutrients tailored to and needed by the individual.

Individualized Vitamins
The individual sends a blood test (blood sample device provided by Baze) which is analyzed in the company's lab. The analysis pinpoints what nutrients in the blood need to be supplemented. The vitamins are customized, filled by prescription and shipped directly to the customer.

Fighting Nutritional Imbalances
Nutritional imbalances are the number one cause of health issues in the US. The company's mission is to address and correct that. Baze has operations in Boston, Berlin, Zurich and San Francisco. They ask their customers to send a blood sample every quarter to keep the dosage optimal. The individual also fills out a questionnaire about their health goals and status.

12. MIT-Harvard Smart Pill: Pill Microneedle

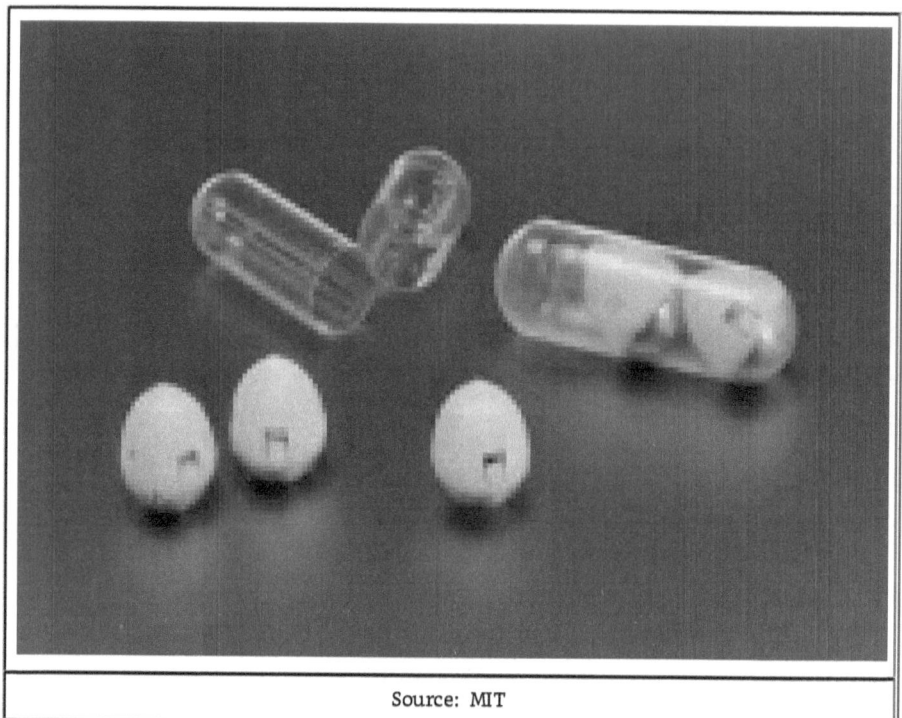

Source: MIT

Radically New Technology Delivers Insulin
Harvard, MIT and insulin manufacturer Novo Nordisk have invented a pill that attaches to the stomach to deliver insulin. For many with Type One diabetes, this could become an attractive alternative to daily injections of insulin by needles. The new capsule is being hailed by global experts as a "radically new technology". The capsule is the size of a blueberry.

Innovative Treatment
The capsule contains a microneedle made of freeze dried insulin. It also contains a tiny stainless steel spring that's held in place by a disc of sugar. The sugar dissolves in the stomach, releasing the spring. The spring pushes the microneedle into the stomach lining. The insulin dissolves into the stomach at a consistent rate. The research team's tests in pigs have proved the capsule to be as effective as daily insulin injections.

More Therapies

The researchers believe the capsule can deliver other therapies, replacing injections and infusions. They are further developing this innovative technology and working to optimize the manufacturing process.

13. Smart Stethoscope With AI: ID's Early Pneumonia

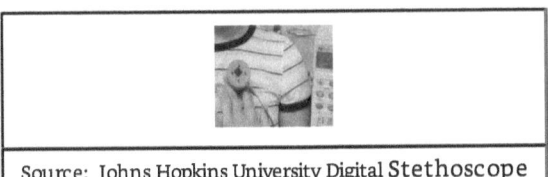

Source: Johns Hopkins University Digital Stethoscope

Artificial Intelligence Smart Device
Johns Hopkins University researchers have developed a smart stethoscope that uses AI to detect early signs of pneumonia. The artificial intelligence powered, smart device listens for specific types of breathing to detect any sign of the disease. If a breathing problem is found, that enables the patient to get much earlier treatment.

Going to Market
The Johns Hopkins team are readying the device for market commercialization. They've created a startup company Sonavi Labs to market the device.

Notable Breakthroughs
This digital stethoscope requires less precise placements on the body. It can pick up significant breathing problems associated with early onslaught pneumonia a bit more widely. It also has strong noise control management that allows it to be used in many, noisy environments.

14. MIT's Remarkable E-Pill: Expands Like a Puffer Fish

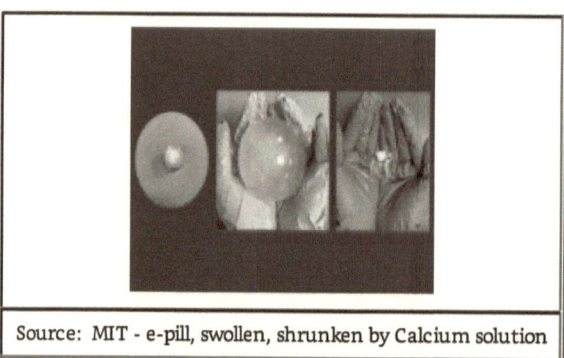

Source: MIT - e-pill, swollen, shrunken by Calcium solution

For Weight Loss and Stomach Monitoring
A team of MIT mechanical engineers have developed an ingestible electronic pill that once in the stomach expands in size like a puffer fish. It rapidly expands in the stomach, has a jello-like consistency and stays in place to take readings overtime. The researchers believe the expanding e-pill can also be used for weight loss.

Sophisticated e-Pill
This is a sophisticated e-pill that swells to the size of a golf ball. The researchers foresee several being ingested to give the stomach the feeling of being full and making it easier to cut calories. The device is composed of two hydrogels - a mixture of water and polymers. It stops in place in the stomach and overcomes the limits of other e-pills that just pass through. It can be equipped with sensors to monitor, for instance, stomach ulcers for 30 days at a time.

Commercializing It
To remove the e-pill, the patient would need to drink a calcium solution that shrinks it and allows it to pass through naturally. It's being lab tested in stomach-like models and the MIT team has plans to commercialize it.

15. Goodbye Toothbrush: France's Fasteesh

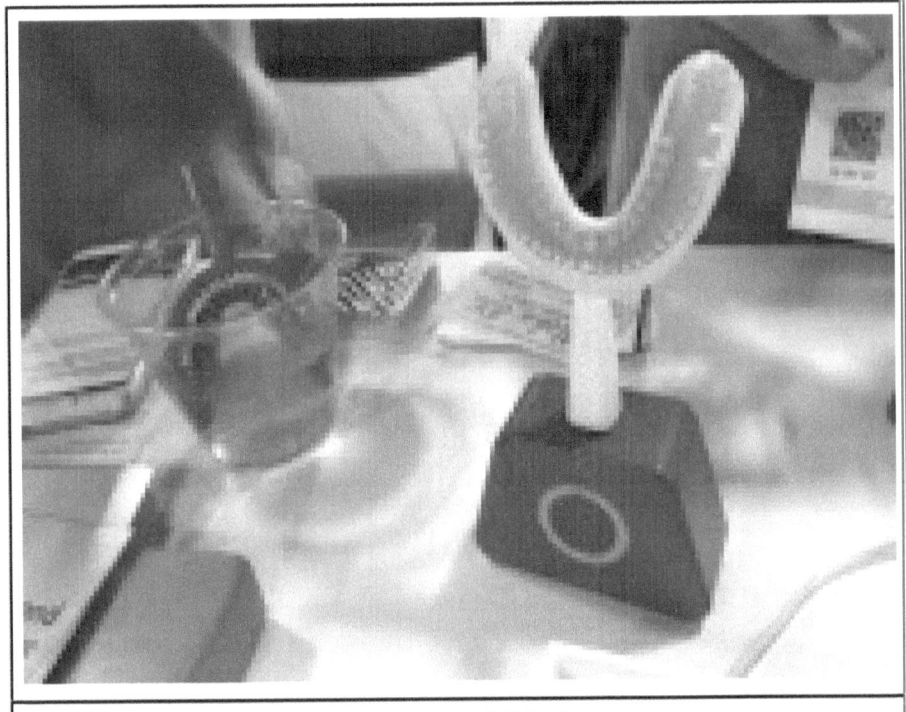

Source: Fasteesh Y-Brush

The Innovative Y-Brush

Imagine cleaning your teeth in ten seconds instead of the several minutes it takes with an ordinary toothbrush. Fasteesh, a French company and creator of the Y-Brush, claims you can achieve the same level of clean with their new product.

Mouthguard

The Y-Brush is a mouth guard that can fit around your upper and lower rows of teeth. The Y-Brush is all nylon bristles placed at 45 degree angles in the mouth guard. It takes just 5 seconds to clean each of the two rows of teeth.

Smaller Sizes for Kids

Awaiting approval by the American Dental Association, it's expected to ship in 2019. The likely price is $125.00. The Y-Brush uses ordinary toothpaste and comes in four sizes, including smaller sizes for children.

16. Smart Patch for Your Health: Patch with Sweat Based Sensors

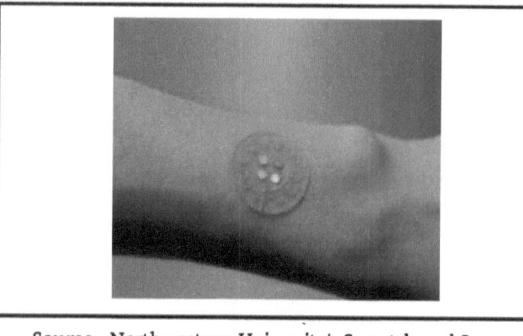

Source: Northwestern University's Sweat-based Sensor

Spots Health Conditions Real-Time

A patch has been developed by bioengineers at Northwestern University that reads your sweat and spots medical conditions. The sweat based sensor provides real-time information on the wearer's levels of chloride, glucose and lactate, sweat rate and pH. The device lets you know if you are dehydrated, lack oxygen, dangerously low on electro-lights, have diabetes or cystic fibrosis.

Next Generation Health Tracker

Today's fitness trackers gather mostly mechanical metrics. A new generation of devices are being developed to access the person's underlying medical conditions. Northwestern's device is a leading example.

Personalized Health Care

Northwestern's device is a personalized approach to fitness and health. It is battery free, wireless and uses sensors and colorimetrics to provide results. To put it simply, the patch has tiny holes where the sweat goes in and moves through microchannels & valves the width of a human hair. The sweat ends up in tiny reservoirs with sensors that react to chemicals in the sweat. It's highly advanced technology. The sweat-based sensors are water-proof, mold to the body and can even be used by swimmers. The readouts can display on a smart phone or even a treadmill.

17. Bot Care-Giving from Samsung

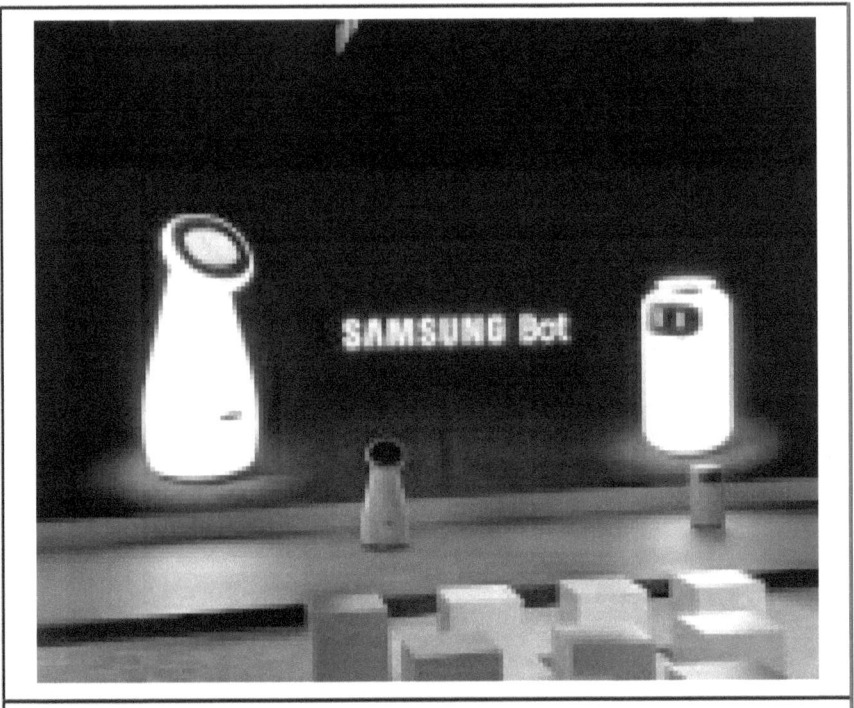

Source: Samsung's Healthcare Bot

Innovative Robotics

Samsung has unveiled what may be the world's most advanced and friendly robot caregiver. Experts are calling it one of the most promising, new developments in robotic innovation in 2019.

Multi-Tasker Bot

This new robot has a great deal of functionality to help in health care delivery for patients. It is equipped with biometric sensors to track your blood pressure and heart rate. It also has a telepresence function to allow your relatives to remind you to take your medicine. And it is also a companion robot to ward off loneliness if you're recovering from or dealing with a long term illness.

Bottom-Line
This is innovative robotic technology that Samsung is still developing but experts say it's already a functional and friendly health care robotic assistant and companion.

18. CES Top Prize: Impossible Burger - "Triumph for Food Engineering"

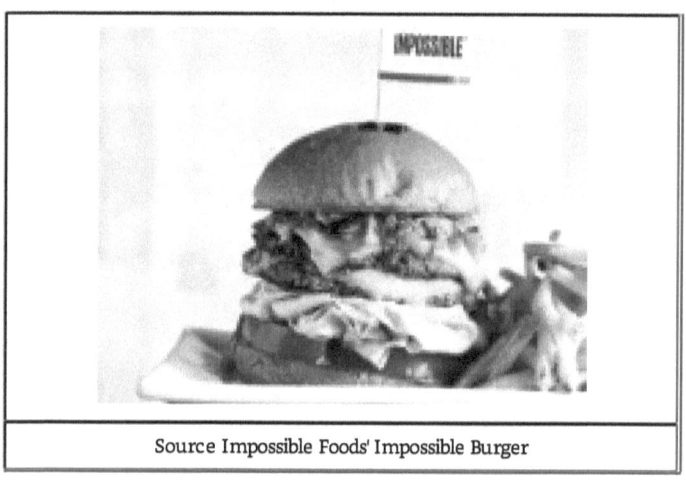

Source Impossible Foods' Impossible Burger

Impossible Burger 2.0 - Innovation Mission Accomplished
Talk about Mission Impossible against 4,400 examples of breakthrough innovation at CES. Impossible Burger, a vegan burger, is the 2019 Consumer Electronics Show's top award winner in innovation. It won "Best in Show", "Best of the Best", "Most Unexpected Product" and "Most Impactful Product". The awards have been re-echoed globally. Digital Trends magazine named the Impossible Burger 2.0 a triumph for food engineering. They're not alone. Engadget called it a vegan burger so tasty that it could eliminate the need for meat. Apparently, the Impossible Burger 2.0 also won the people's choice award at the 2019 CES in Las

Vegas.

Impossible Foods

The noteworthy burger is made by Impossible Foods, a startup based in Redwood City, CA, founded by Dr. Patrick Brown, Professor Emeritus at Stanford. The burger is a plant based meat replacement that's meatier. They use soy instead of wheat to take on various forms of vegan ground meat including for burgers, lasagna and tacos. In the US, the vegan burgers are rolled out in 20 high end restaurants. Impossible Foods' 5,000 partner restaurants are putting it on their vegan menus. Beyond that, it's available in Hong Kong and Macau.

2019: Year of the Vegan

The Economist calls 2019 "The Year of the Vegan." Impossible Burger 2.0 is being called an instant success. They are now targeting the Holy Grail of Vegan - a tasty vegan steak. And Dr. Brown is scaling up his business fast.

19. My Brain, My Computer: Elon Musk's Neuralink

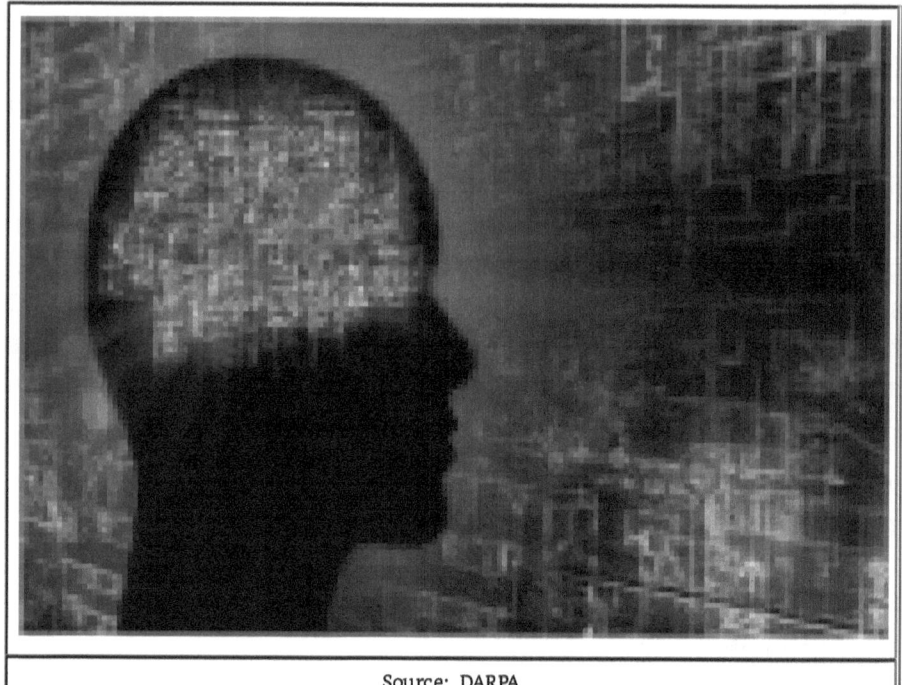

Source: DARPA

Musk Believes You'll Be Able to Connect Your Brain to Computers in 10 Years

Elon Musk is an extraordinary innovator, entrepreneur and engineer. He founded and is CEO of Tesla, SpaceX, the Boring Company and Neuralink. With Neuralink, he's betting that you'll be able to connect your brain to computers to enhance your intelligence in ten years.

Neuralink

His vision is the development of ultra high bandwidth brain-machine interfaces to connect humans with machines. Neuralink is developing the interface technology. Musk says this will be done by connecting computer electrodes to neurons in your brain. It would consist of a chip and according to Musk "a bunch of tiny wires implanted in your skull." He believes it can be done. So, does the US Defense Department's Advanced Research Projects Agency - DARPA - which is also working on developing the technology to make it happen.

Building the Start-Up Company

Neuralink is based in San Francisco. On the website, Musk is recruiting scientists and engineers. The visionary engineer argues that the way we interface with our phones, computers and watches is the beginning of brain-computer interfacing. He calls the devices "a tertiary digital layer on your cognition."

20. NASA Discovery: Parts of DNA Can Form in Space

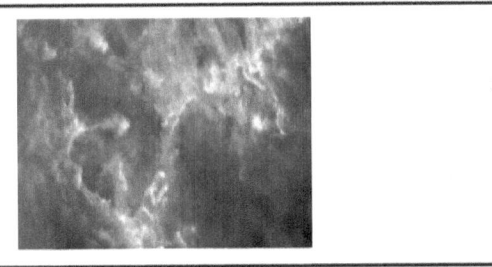

Source: European Space Agency Shot of Eagle Nebula - Frigid & Radiation Rich

Stuff of Life

Parts of DNA, the stuff of life, can form in space. NASA scientists have made deoxyribose, the sugar that is the backbone of DNA, under space-like conditions. In a lab, they blasted ice with radiation and discovered 2-deoxyribose. Their innovation and findings are published in the journal Nature Communications.

NASA Research

NASA astrochemist Michael Nuevo says their research shows that the process of DNA formation can happen anywhere in our galaxy. It suggests that the stuff of life could have been delivered to earth from elsewhere.

Process

The scientists cooled frozen water and frozen methane to -260 degrees. Inside a vacuum, they blasted it with ultraviolet light mimicking conditions in interstellar clouds. Warming the irradiated ice simulated what occurs when a young star is born. The scientists identified 2-deoxyribose in the ice.

Asteroid Missions

NASA and Japan have two asteroid missions going on. They will bring back samples. And the scientists hope to search for deoxyribose in them.

21. eBandage Accelerates Healing: Innovation from a Global Scientific Team

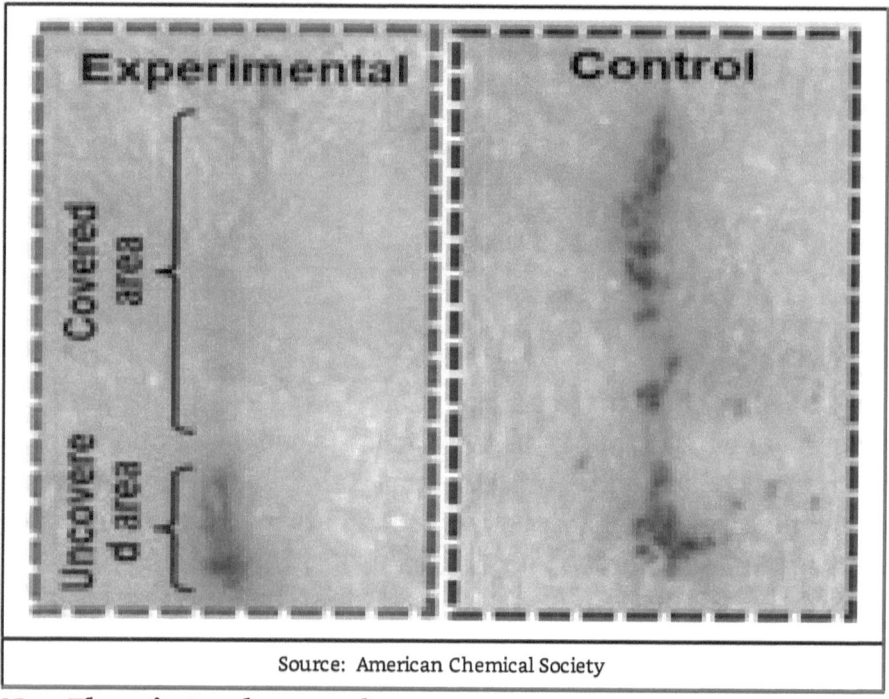

Source: American Chemical Society

New Electric Bandage Heals

It's a self-powered, electric bandage that generates an electric field over an injury. It dramatically reduces the healing time. The innovation comes from a global team of scientists - China's University of Electronic Science & Technology and the University of Wisconsin.

Healing Electric Field

They've created a flexible, self-powered bandage that converts normal skin movements into a therapeutic electric field.

Dramatic Results

The power comes from a wearable nano-generator. It converts normal movements into small electrical pulses. The current flows to two electrodes placed on either side of a wound. That creates a small electric field over the wound. The results are dramatic. Wounds covered by the eBandage closed in 3 days. Those without the eBandage averaged 12 days.

22. Ingestible Electronic Pill, Smartphone Controlled

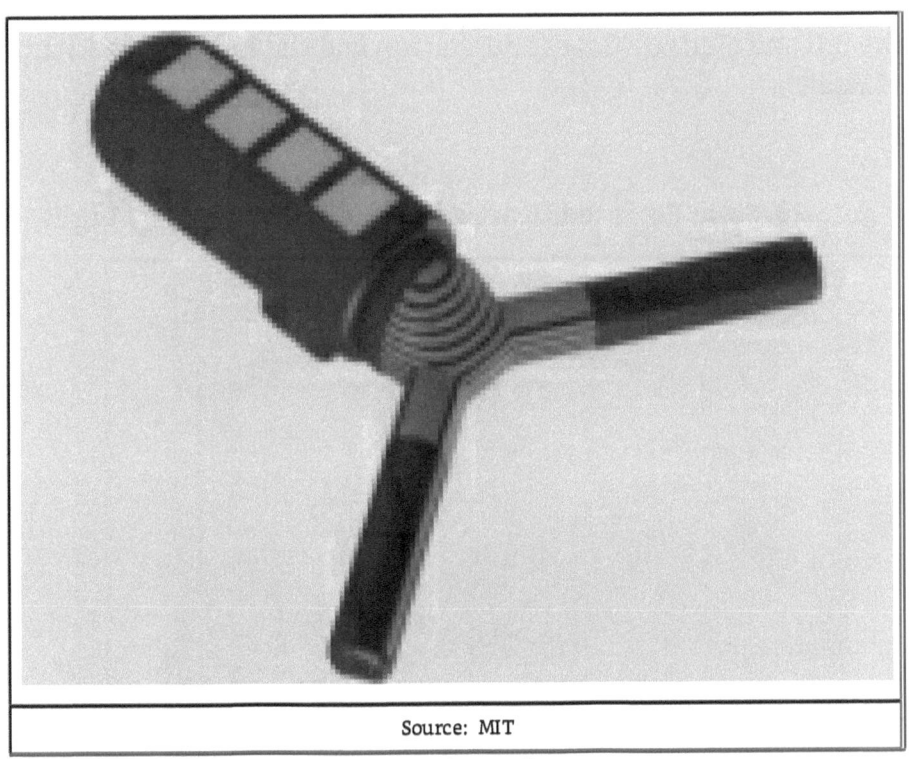

Source: MIT

Medical Innovation on the Cutting Edge

MIT scientists, along with Draper Lab and Brigham & Women's Hospital researchers, have done it again. They've created an ingestible electronic pill that's controlled by Bluetooth wireless technology. The device can be customized to deliver drugs, include sensors to monitor gastric conditions or do both. It's cutting edge ingestible technology that the team produces by 3D printing.

Smart Phone Controlled

It can reside in the stomach for a month. All the while responding to instructions from a user's smartphone and transmitting information. The scientists say it can be used to treat a variety of diseases by delivering drugs particularly over a long time period. It can also be customized to spot infections, allergic reaction and specifically target and calibrate therapy deliveries. And it can provide the information it's collecting to the patient's and doctor's smart phones. This breakthrough innovation was funded by the Bill and Melinda Gates Foundation and the National Institute of Health.

23. Solar Powered Hearts: Pacemaker Powered by Light

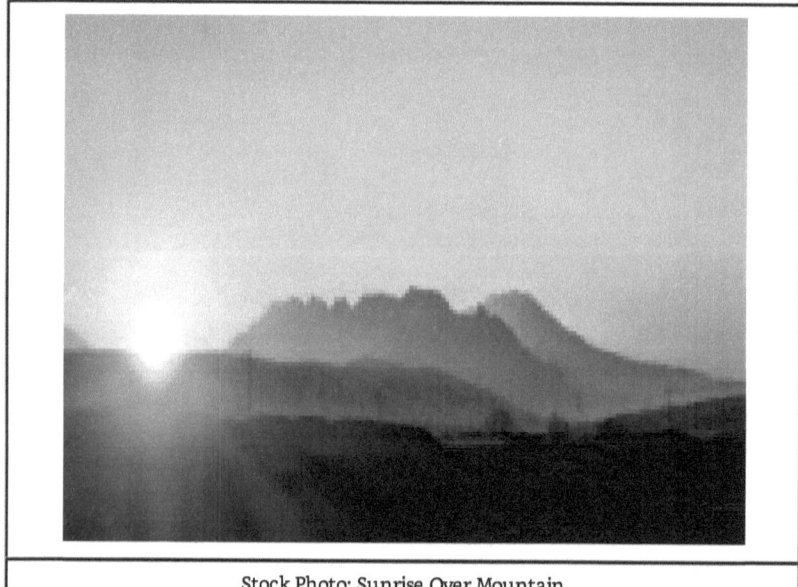

Stock Photo: Sunrise Over Mountain

Solar Energy Heart Beats

This is a tiny, solar cell that keeps the heart beating. In fact, it seems to teach the heart how to beat. It's an innovation that may lead to heart pacemakers powered by light. It's new innovation invented by scientists at the University of Chicago. It's totally new and quite exciting.

Specs

They've created a flexible mesh from silicon that wraps around the heart. They threaded nanowires across it to connect with cardiac cells. When activated by light, it creates a tiny electrochemical effect that stimulates the heart muscles in a unique way. A small optical beam scans the heart area with a laser. Each flash activates the cells, causing the heart to beat at the rate of the light.

Breakthrough Medical Innovation

This research has been published in the journal Proceedings of the National Academy of Sciences. The researchers used a device they developed to stimulate neurons and retrofitted it. They made the mesh thinner to wrap around the heart. The method is in the early stages of development.

24. Genetics Behind Active and Sedentary Lifestyles: Oxford University

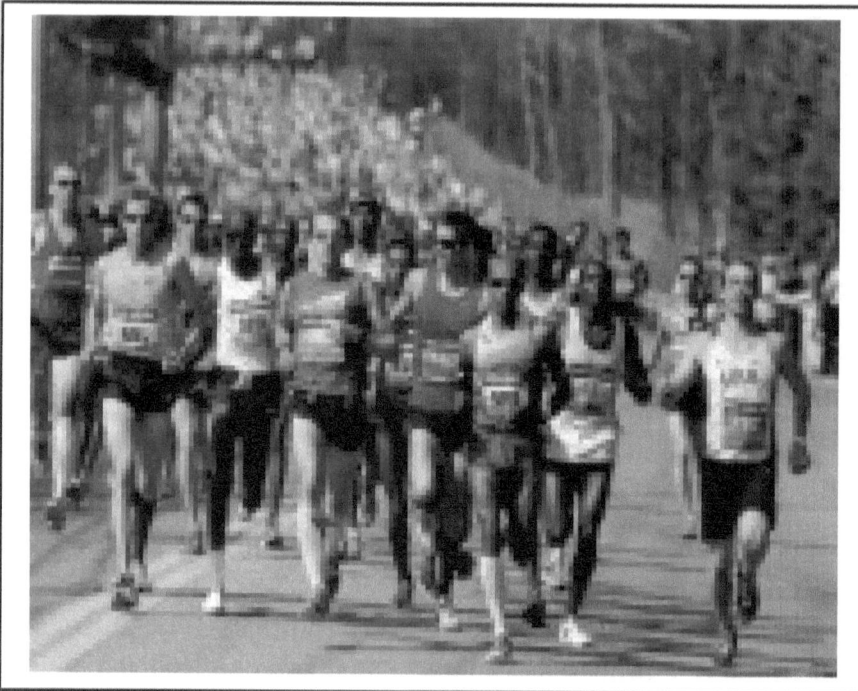
Source: Photo of Boston Marathon

Causes & Consequences of Physical Inactivity

New research shows there's a complex genetic basis to even some of the most fundamental human functions like moving, resting and sleeping. Scientists at Oxford University in the UK have discovered the amount of time that an individual sleeps, moves and rests is determined in part by their genes. They're exploring the causes and consequences of physical inactivity. For example, they hope to determine if inactivity is a cause or a consequence of obesity.

One of the Most Detailed Studies on Lifestyle

91,105 UK Biobank participants were actively monitored. Machine learning models identified active and sedentary lifestyles.

Important Outcomes

Their analysis revealed 14 genetic regions related to activity - 7 totally new to science. The research was published in Nature

Communication. It shows that physical activity casually lowers your blood pressure. It provides a better understanding of sleep, physical activity and their health consequences. It is important medical discovery and innovation being spearheaded by a multi-disciplinary group of scientists.

25. DARPA's Breakthrough for Depression Treatment

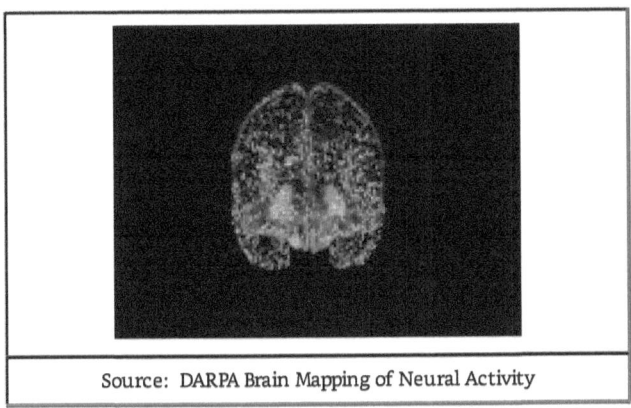

Source: DARPA Brain Mapping of Neural Activity

Could "Radically Improve Treatment"

A team of researchers working for the US Defense Department's Advanced Research Projects Agency DARPA say they've made a series of breakthrough discoveries that may radically improve the treatment of depression, anxiety and other mood disorders.

The researchers are from the University of California San Francisco, Massachusetts General Hospital and the University of Southern California. From their research, they have

- Detailed a new technology that analyzes and decodes recorded neural signals to predict changes in mood
- Identified a sub-network of the brain that contributes to low moods
- Detailed how they used an open-loop neural stimulator to relieve symptoms of moderate to severe depression.

This DARPA program is called SUBNETS. It's focused on improving understanding of the subnetworks of the brain.

26. New 10 Minute Test Detects Cancer

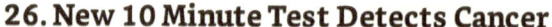

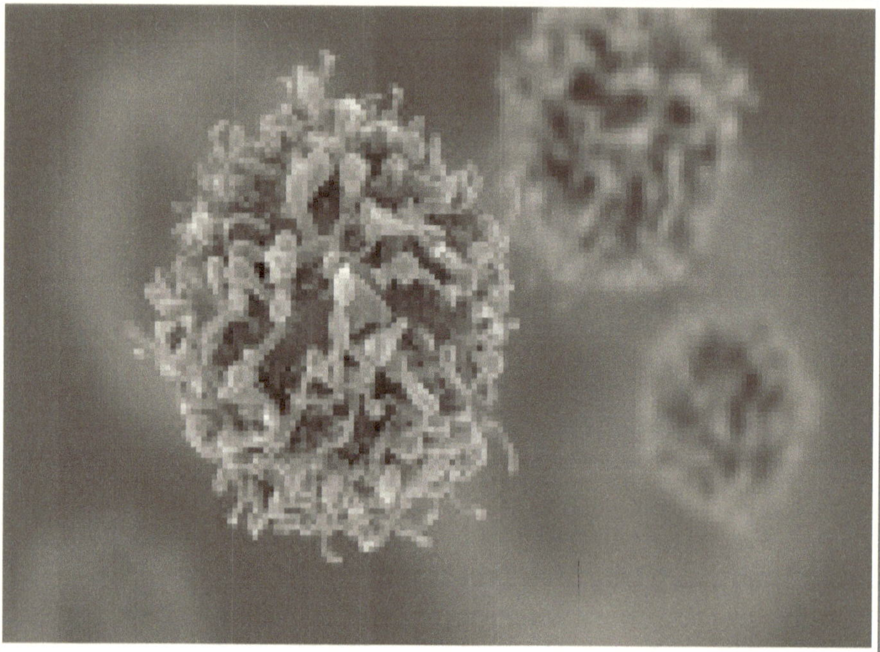

Source: Cancer Cells

Noninvasive, Inexpensive, Universal Cancer Test
The 10 minute test can detect cancer anyplace in the body. The test was developed after scientists at the University of Queensland discovered that cancer forms a unique DNA structure when placed in water. The test works by identifying the presence of that structure.

DNA
Cancerous DNA molecules form entirely different 3D nanostructures than normal DNA molecules do. That discovery enabled the scientists to innovate a new, noninvasive approach to detect cancer in any tissue including blood.

Easy Test

They say their test is inexpensive, portable and possibly may be performed with a mobile phone. It's believed the test could detect cancer much earlier, which is a key to successful outcomes. Their work was published in the journal Nature Communications.

27. Israeli Breath Test Detects Disease: SNIFFPHONES

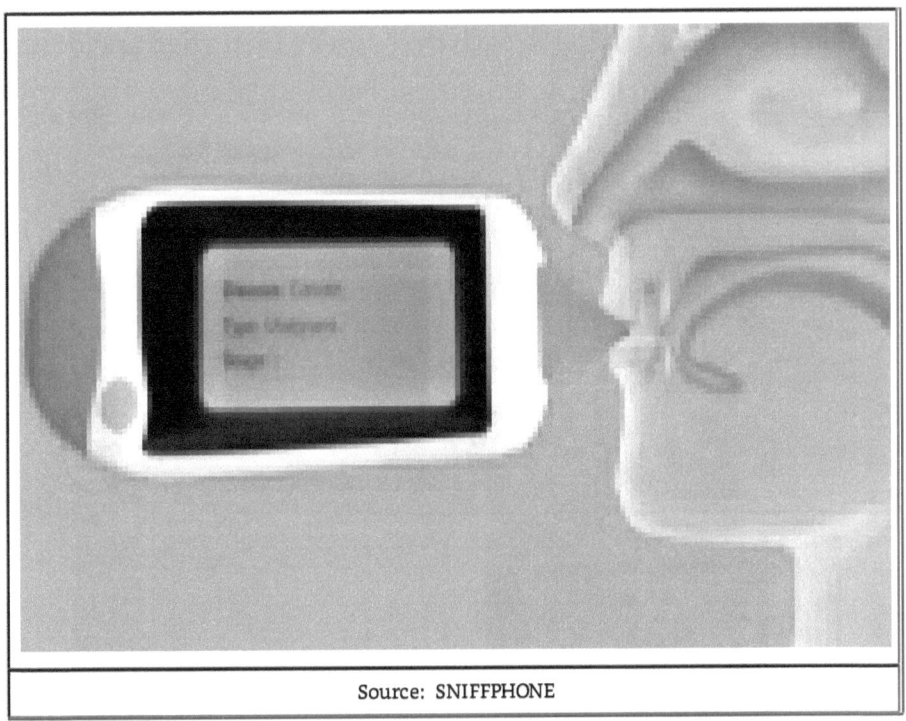

Source: SNIFFPHONE

Breakthrough Innovation from Israel

It's called the SNIFFPHONE. It uses nanotechnology sensors to analyze particles in the breath and pinpoints evidence of disease. The diseases include certain types of cancers, pulmonary disease and the early stages of neurodegenerative diseases.

Putting a Micro-Chip into a Breathalyzer-Like Device

This device has been awarded the European Commission's Innovation Prize. The recipient is Israeli Professor Hossam Haick of the Wolfson faculty of Chemical Engineering at the Technion -Israel Institute of Technology. The scientist says this is all about humanity and our digital future. He was cited by the Commission as the most innovative scientist achieving an idea in electronic systems.

Microchips and Biomarkers

The Israeli team placed a microchip into a breathalyzer-like device to diagnose unique fingerprints of disease. These are biomarkers of disease on the breath that can be identified and could save lives.

28. Running a Marathon Blind: World History Made in NYC

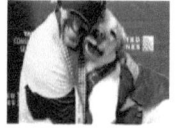

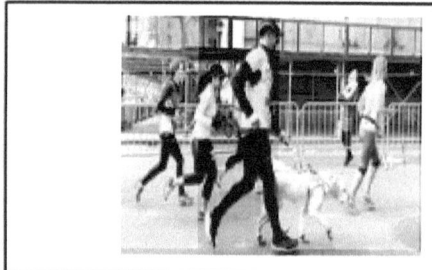

Source: Thomas Panek and Gus at NYC Marathon

Blind Runner Completes Race with his Guide Dog Gus

Thomas Panek became the first runner to complete the NYC Half Marathon with no sight. He crossed the finish line with his long time guide dog Gus. Panek lost his sight 25 years ago but he never lost his love of running. At first frightened to run, he started running again being guided by human volunteers. But, being tied to another person eliminated the independence of running for him. So, he tried an innovative approach - running with his guide dog. He made history at the NYC Half Marathon, finishing the race with his long time guide dog Gus with no human assistance.

CEO/Entrepreneur Panek and His Team of 3 Labs

The athlete is CEO of Guiding Eyes for the Blind, a nonprofit that provides "superbly bred and trained dogs" for blind and visually impaired, free of charge. For the NYC race, Mr. Panek actually used his trio of three Lab guide dogs - Westley, Waffle and Gus, each for a third of the race. Gus took the runner to the finish line. Mission accomplished, so Gus retired. The dogs wore special harnesses and running boots to protect their paws. They keep the blind runner safe by spotting any obstacles and impediments in his way.

Innovation and Entrepreneurship

Panek has been running with his guide dogs for many years. In 2015, he established the Running Guides Program which trains dogs to support runners. He's completed more than 20 marathons with human volunteers as guides. He says he appreciated their support but missed the independence of just running with his guide dogs. At the NYC Half Marathon, he accomplished his goal of showing the world how to run a marathon without sight, confident in the guide dogs by your side. The team finished the race in 2 hours & 21 minutes.

29. OnMed Telemedicine Booths

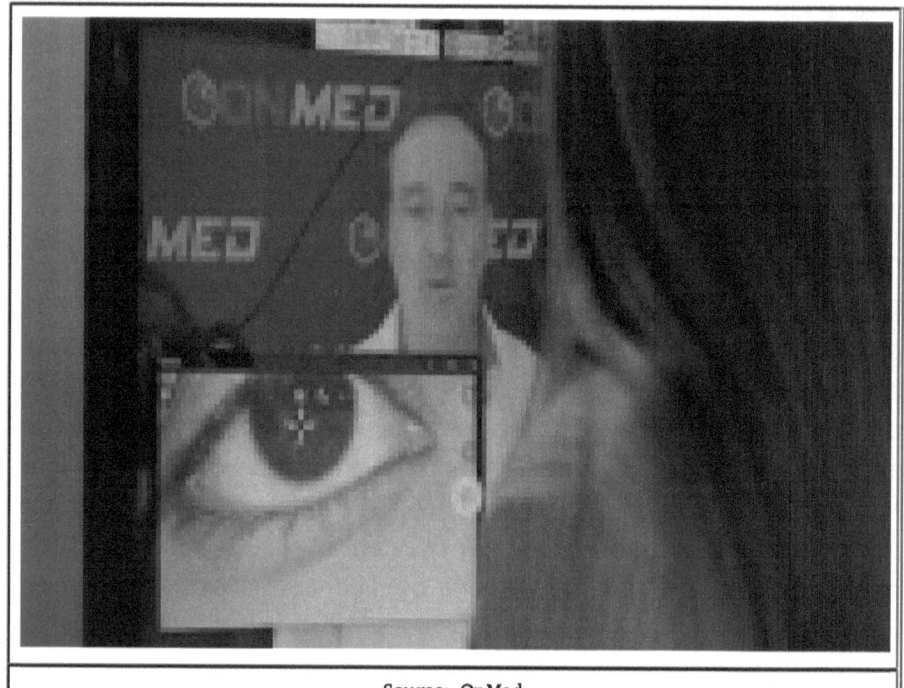

Source: OnMed

Innovation and Technology at the Cutting Edge of Health Care
The concept is drawn from the public accessibility of old, land line telephone booths. But the application is new, innovative and exciting for telemedicine. OnMed's Telemedicine Booths have the potential to make health care much more accessible, affordable and convenient for the general public. The company will roll out the first stations in Mississippi in 2019.

Six Years Under Development
OnMed is a Clearwater, FL based company. It's been developing this "doctor in a booth" innovative technology concept for six years. The small booth, OnMed Station is equipped with a lot of sensors, video and audio technologies, including facial recognition technology to ensure privacy. Doctor and patient can communicate in real time and data can be transmitted to the doctor from the booth. The data includes weight, height, blood pressure and blood oxygen levels. The system can even provide a thermal

image of the person's body and send it to the doctor for medical review. It even has an HD camera to look down a patient's throat.

New Health Care Innovation

After the data is gathered, the station can dispense medicine from its onboard supply or print a prescription via the online doctor. OnMed guarantees their doctors are board certified. They also guarantee patient confidentiality and security and a UV lighting system to sanitize the booths between visits. This unstaffed booth is designed for use by health care systems, employers and government organizations to facilitate access to busy ER departments. The company is targeting this new health care access system at airports, rural locations, campuses and worksites for 24/7 healthcare.

30. AI Hearing Aid: Evoke's Machine Learning Technology

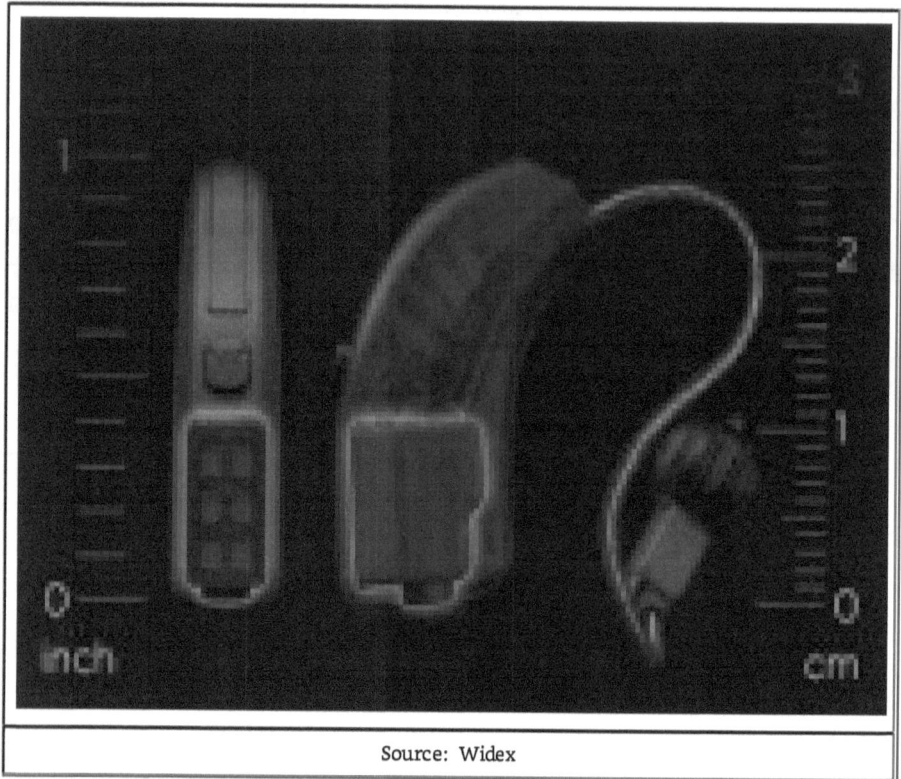

Source: Widex

Very Smart Hearing Aids
It's called Evoke. It's an AI enhanced hearing aid just developed that's state of the art. The smart device uses machine learning to optimize sound quality for the listener. With millions of people globally having impaired hearing, this new innovation has great humanitarian potential. This new technology was introduced at 2019 CES by Widex. The company calls it high definition hearing.

SoundSense AI Technology
The device's AI SoundSense technology pulls in real time data and uses it to adjust volume and customize settings for the individual. It's a battery-free hearing device.

Widex Energy Cell
Evoke is powered by Widex's Energy cell that combines oxygen and methanol and lasts for 24 hours. The recharge takes only 20

seconds and it's good to go for another day.

31. New Motion Capture Suit: For Athletes and Others, Full Body 3D Motion Tracking

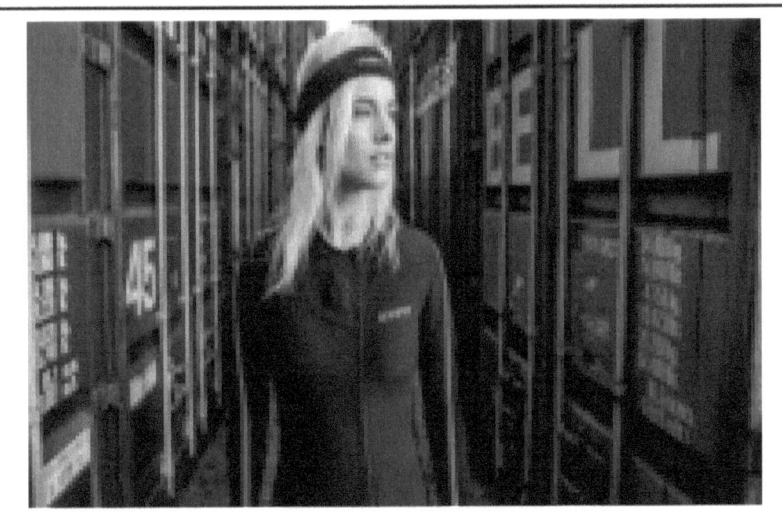

Source: XSENS Motion Tracking Bodysuit

XSENS Innovation from the Netherlands

XSENS, based in The Netherlands, is a leading innovator in 3D motion tracking technologies. Their latest technology offers full body, 3D movement analysis by wireless data capture. They've introduced two new systems.

MVN Awinda

Their new MVN Awinda offers a full-body motion analysis that's optimized for sports and ergonomic uses. It deploys 17 wireless trackers wrapped around the performer such as in a headband, wrist, arm and leg bands. Movement data from them is transmitted up to 60 feet indoors and 150 feet outdoors to a backpack called an Awinda station where the data is streamed live or recorded.

Full Bodysuit

Another new product is the MVN Link bodysuit. It is a lycra body-suit with wireless trackers built-in. It comes in 5 sizes and has a wireless range for data transmission of 150 feet indoors and 450 feet outdoors. The bodysuit transmits the data to a central data link that resends or streams the data. This is new technology to help athletes, assembly line workers and perhaps those undergoing physical rehabilitation to rebuild their limbs.

32. AI Beanie: Smart Hat to Helmet When Needed

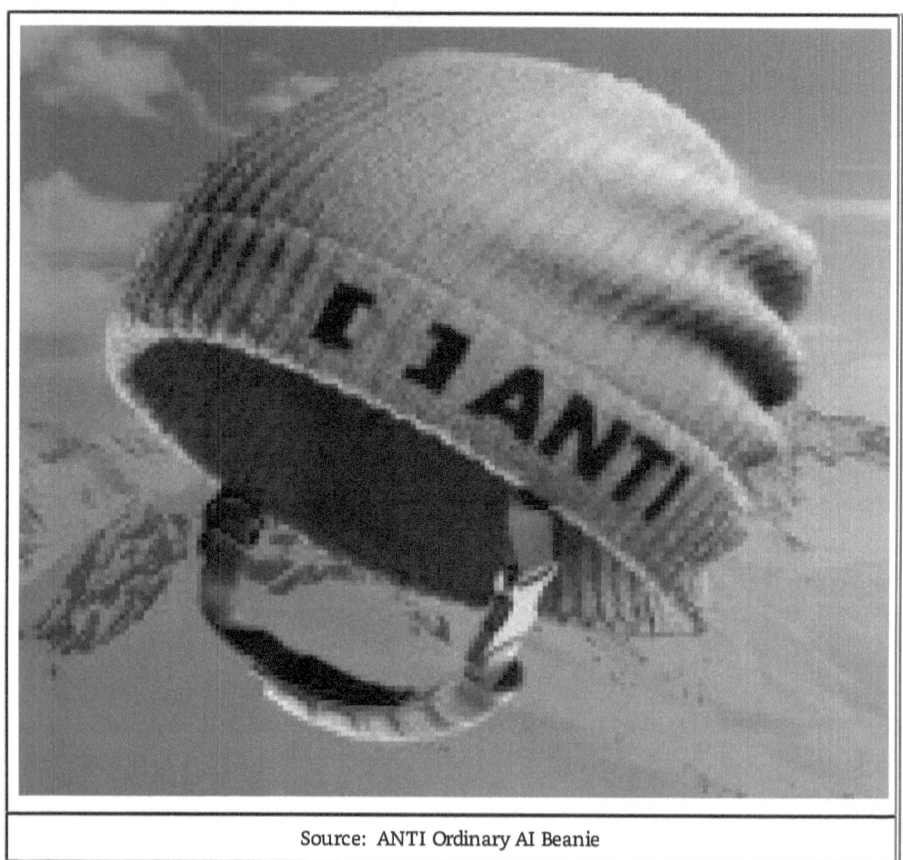

Source: ANTI Ordinary AI Beanie

AI Shifts Hat from Soft to Helmet-Like Protection
The company ANTI Ordinary says this hat is as safe as a helmet and you'll find it your most comfortable helmet ever. It's called

the AI Beanie and has soft, Merino wool knitted lining and a moisture repellent acrylic outer layer. What is between those two layers is the differentiator.

Non-Newtonian Fluids - Not Your Ordinary Hat
What is between the two layers is the company's proprietary blend of non-Newtonian fluids. The fluid particles remain soft and flexible in slow motion and become much harder when impacted. The inner layer of the hat becomes stiff enough to exceed safety standards while flexible enough to pack in a backpack and easily fit the contours of the head. It's deliverable in October 2019, priced at $125.00 and seems targeted particularly at outdoor winter sports.

33. 3D Bioprinter: Personalized Wound Healing That's Mobile

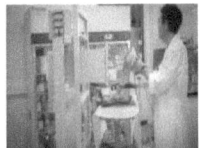

Source: Wake Forrest University

Medicine on the Cutting Edge
This is remarkable innovation. Millions of Americans suffer from non-healing wounds. A team at Wake Forrest University has developed a 3D bioprinter that can selectively layer skin cells to heal a large wound or burn. The process is personalized to the patient. The bioprinter is filled with the patient's own skin cells.

Several Firsts
There are a number of firsts involved in this innovation. The bioprinter is mobile and can be wheeled directly to the patient's bed. It enables on-site management of large wounds by 3D laser scanning and measuring them in order to deposit cells directly where they're needed to create new skin. It selectively layers in two types of cells. Fibroplasts are placed on the deepest part of

the wound and keratinocytes on top.

Mimics Natural Healing

The 3D bioprinter and the healing process it delivers replicate natural tissue and promotes healing. The team has successfully demonstrated proof of concept and now will take it through human trials.

34. Smart Lighter to Quit Smoking: Slighter

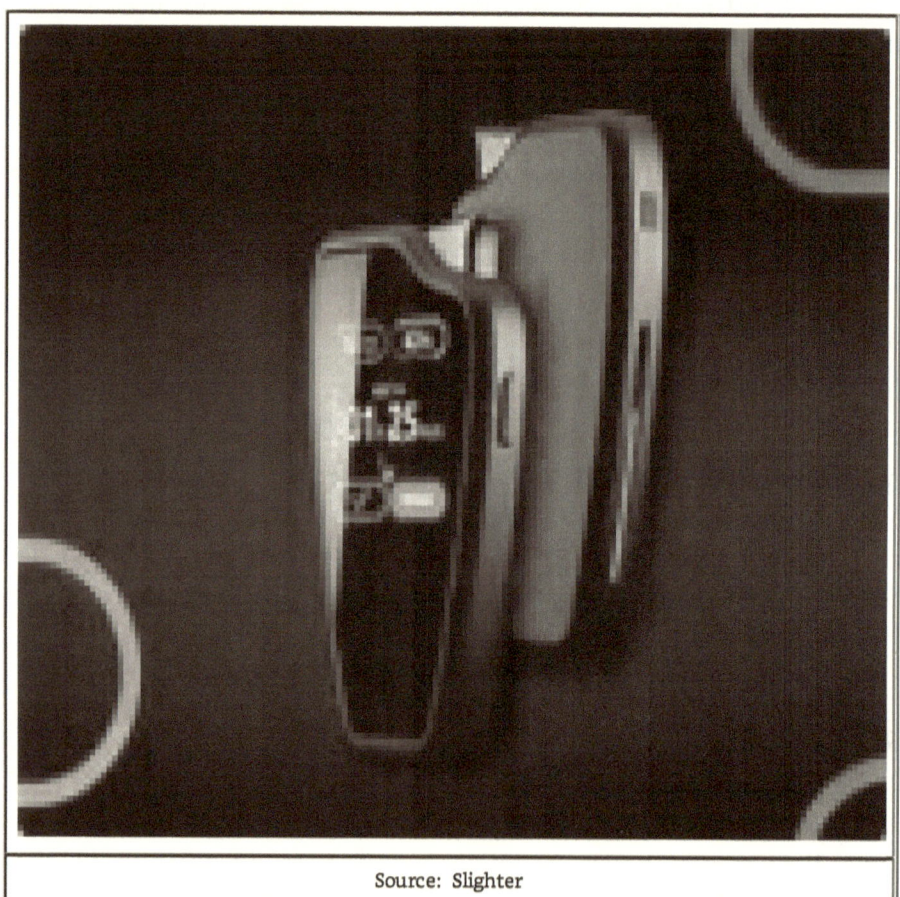

Source: Slighter

Innovation from Lebanon

Slighter is the latest, smart lighter that can help you quit smoking one cigarette at a time. The company is based in Lebanon. Their product offers a new way to quit smoking. It learns from your habits. It calculates how frequently you smoke and when you do so. It uses the data to customize a plan for each smoker.

Elegantly Simple Innovation that's Easy to Use

There's a lot of innovation and ingenuity in this smart lighter concept. It sometimes, on purpose, won't light up to help the smoker cut cigarettes eventually down to zero. The price is $129. It will start shipping in the summer 2019. The French National Cancer Institute plans to do a trial run with it.

Communicates and Calculates

You can communicate and share the data on your progress to quit smoking on a phone app. The device also tells you how much money you've saved as you reach your quit smoking goals. Interesting and innovative technology innovation developed in Lebanon.

35. Healthifyme: Digital Weight Loss Platform

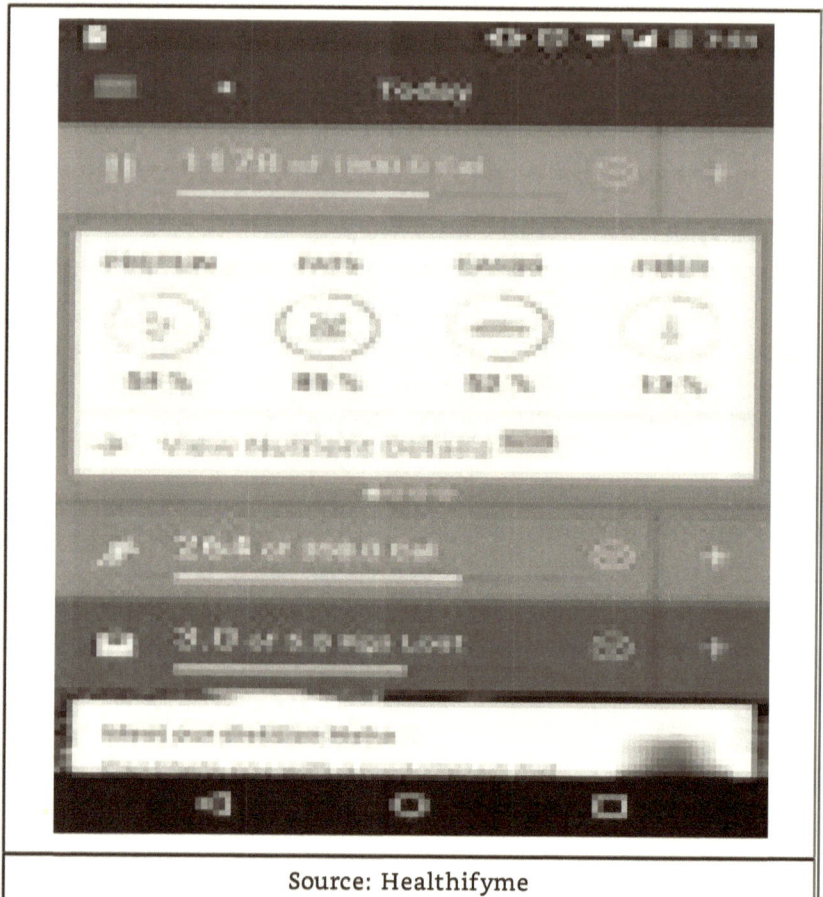

Source: Healthifyme

Coaching from the Cloud

Based in India, Healthifyme is a digital weight loss platform that provides fitness and weight services. Developed for Android and iOS platforms, the app provides calorie and water tracking and on the cloud fitness coaching. The company is gearing up to launch Ria 2.0, its personal AI assistant that can make dietary recommendations and calculate calories on the spot. The app has a paid version where, for instance, you can chat with nutritionists and health coaches to help maximize your results.

Global Expansion

The innovative technology company is expanding globally. It's in Malaysia, the United Arab Emirates, Singapore and planning to enter Saudi Arabia soon. The device takes into account age, weight, goals, pre-existing medical conditions and recommends customized "smart meal plans". The company plans to integrate Ria with Google Assistant and Alexa this year.

36. World's First Vaccine to Save Bees: Critical to World Food Supplies

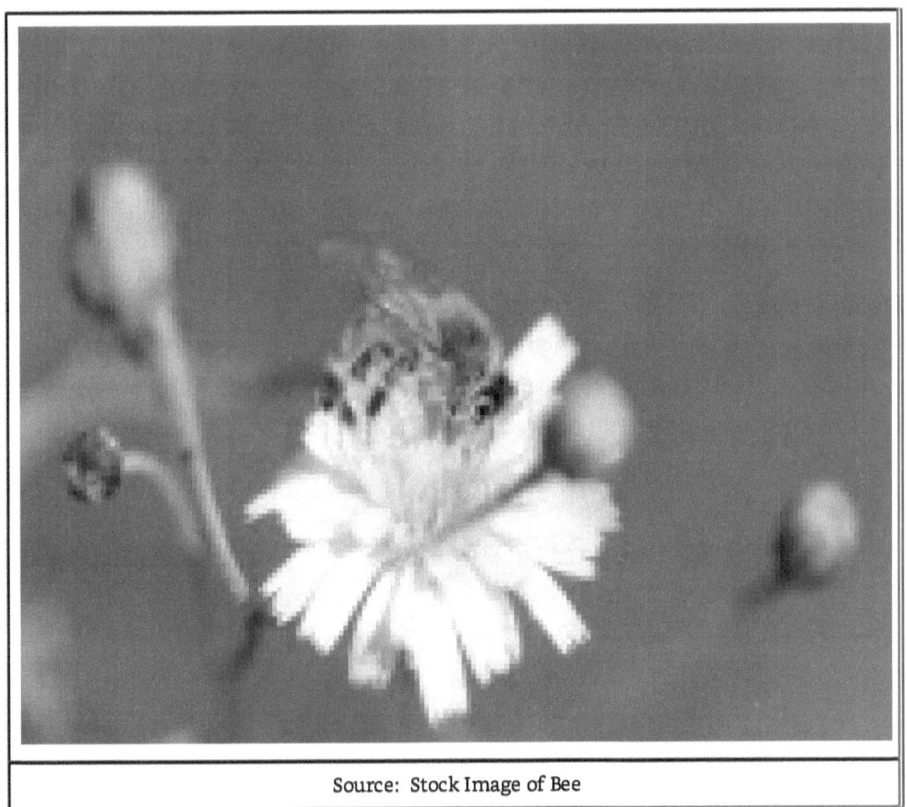

Source: Stock Image of Bee

Medical Innovation Breakthrough from Finland

Bees are vital to the production of global food supplies. They help fertilize 3 out of 4 crops globally. They do so by transferring pollen from male to female flowers. Bees are being wiped out by disease. Scientists in Finland have innovated the world's first vaccine to protect bees against disease.

49

Drastic Bee Population Decline

There has been a drastic decline in bee numbers that could cause a global food crisis. The bees have been dying from what's called "colony collapse disorder", a mysterious bee epidemic world-wide. A United Nations study indicates that 40% of the world's bees and butterflies face extinction. Scientists warn that will result in higher food prices and food shortages.

Medical Innovation Breakthrough

The new vaccine was developed by scientists at Helsinki University. It works by giving the bees resistance to fight microbial diseases that can be fatal to the pollinators. The vaccine involves a protein and certain bacteria that pass on immunity to the next generation through the queen bee. The queen receives the vaccine by a sugar cube.

Next Steps

For the scientists who innovated this breakthrough vaccine, they now face customary regulatory hurdles to clear. They think it will take 4 to 5 years to reach market.

37. From Tasmanian Devils Cancer Cure: Certain Genes Shrink Tumors

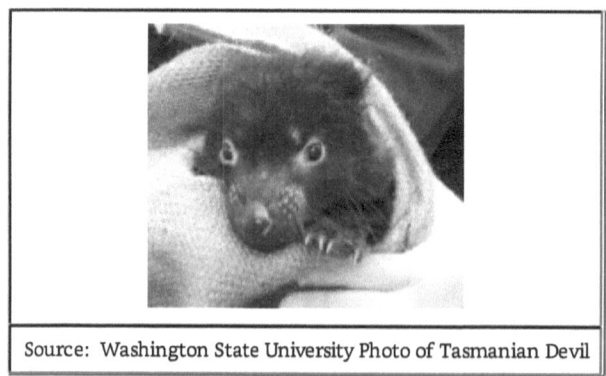

Source: Washington State University Photo of Tasmanian Devil

Washington State University Innovative Cancer Research

Scientists at Washington State University have discovered genes and genetic mutations that appear to shrink deadly cancer tumors in Tasmanian devils. This finding could have important implications for treating cancer in humans and other mammals.

Cancer Fighting Genes Leading to Drug Creation
The WSU scientists say some of the genes that they believe trigger tumor regression in the devils are also in humans. This could lead to the development of drugs that shrink and potentially decimate tumors in humans.

A Species Plagued by Cancer
The devils are the largest carnivorous marsupial and found only in Tasmania. A deadly, facial tumor disease has pushed the devils to near extinction. 80% of the population is gone. An international team of scientists, led by WSU, found some of the animals are developing genetic resistance to the disease that shrinks the tumors and ends the cancer. Their findings have been published in the journal Genome Biology and Evolution.

38. Your Brain Predicts the Future: Uses Two Clocks to Anticipate

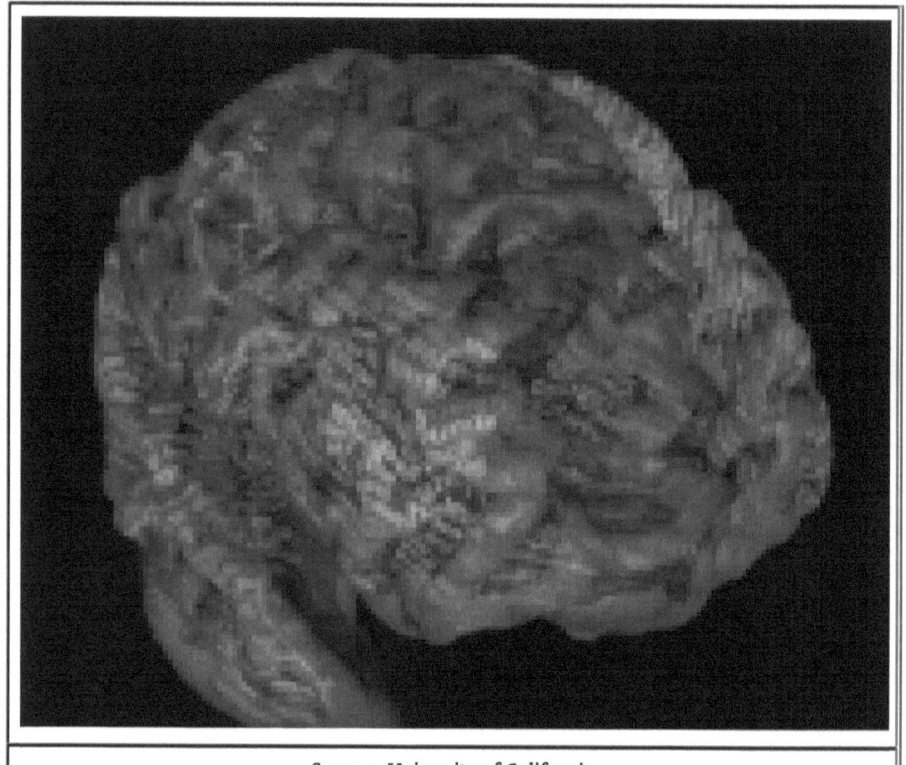

Source: University of California

Innovative Research - University of California - Berkeley
It's called anticipatory timing by the brain. And it's a two barreled system. One type of timing relies on memories from past experience. A second type is based on rhythm. They work together. An example is putting your foot on the car's gas pedal as the light starts turning from red to green. Berkeley neuroscientists have discovered that in music, sports, speech and other activities we calculate movements in two parts of the brain.

Brain Timekeepers
The neural networks supporting these timekeepers are split between two different parts of the brain. The scientists discovered that timing isn't a unified process. Their research has documented that there are two different ways we make temporal decisions and they are dependent on different parts of the brain.

Your Brain Actively Anticipating the Future
Berkeley scientists have provided a new perspective through their innovative research on how we calculate when to make a move. According to lead author/UC Berkeley neuroscientist Richard Ivry, together these brain systems allow us not just to exist in the moment but also actively anticipate the future.

Relevancy to Brain Disorders
This breakthrough research was published in the Proceedings of the National Academy of Science Journal. It holds particular relevancy to helping those with Parkinson's disease and cerebella disorders at the outset of this great research.

39. Heart Benefits from Strength Training Exercise

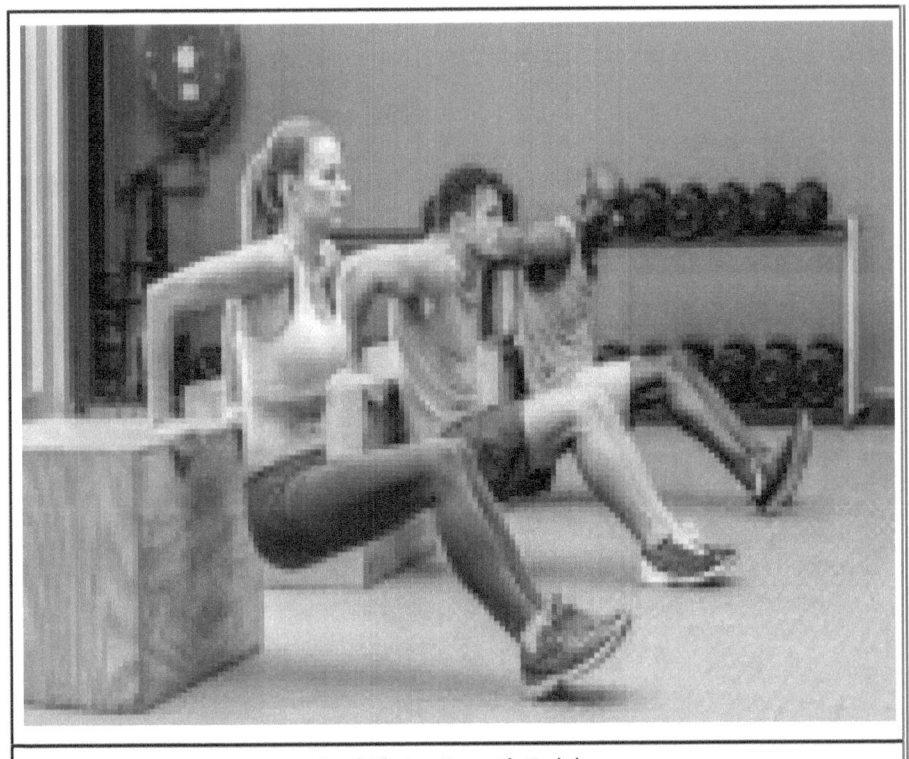

Stock Photo: Strength Training

New Research

The American College of Cardiology reports that static exercise activity like strength training is good and better for your heart. It has stronger results for reducing heart disease risk than dynamic exercise activity like cycling, running and walking.

Results

The results were presented at the LCC Latin America Conference 2018 in Lima, Peru. More than 4,000 American adults were tracked and analyzed on their exercise routines. The research concludes that all types of physical activity and exercise are good for the heart. But static activities, like aerobics and strength training, even in small amounts, proved to be the most beneficial.

Your Takeaways

The bottom-line from this research is that all exercise works. Static and dynamic work separately, they work together but static exercise stands out as the most beneficial in preventing heart disease.

40. Top Scientists Demand Insecticide Ban: Brain Development At Risk

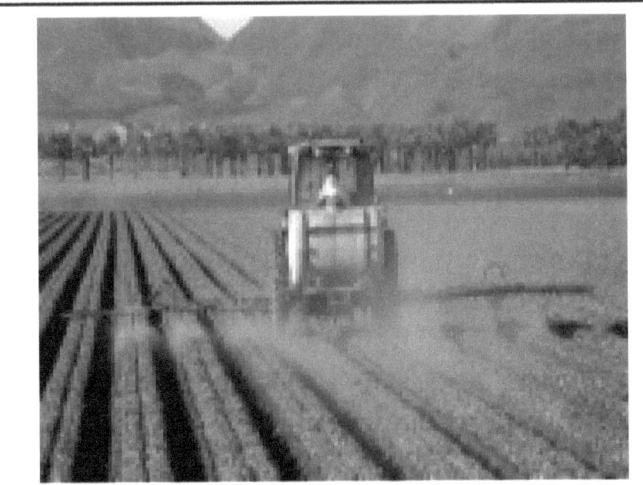

Source: Stock Photo Pesticide Spraying

Widely Used Organophosphates Cause Big Risk to Early Brain Development

This breakthrough research on insecticides widely used on farms, in malls and schools is from the University of California Davis. The scientists have overwhelming evidence that prenatal exposure to common insecticides known as organophosphates puts children at risk for neurodevelopmental disorders. The scientists are calling for immediate government action to phase the chemicals out. Their scientific review and demand for action was published in PLOS Medicine.

Low Exposure to the Chemicals Leads to Lower IQ

The study found "compelling evidence" that even low exposure in pregnant women to the organophosphate pesticides is associated with lower IQs and difficulties in learning, memory and attention in their children. The scientists are implicating the entire class of organophosphate pesticides.

Widely Used on Farms and in Public Places

It's important to know that these pesticides originated as nerve gases and weapons of war. Today they have been converted into use to control insects on farms, schools, shopping malls and golf courses. Their essential mission remains the same: they kill insects by blocking their nerve signals.

Widespread Contact

The vast majority of Americans come in contact with these chemicals. They're in the food we eat, the water we drink and the air we breathe. Some governmental limits on their use have been put in place. But, the U-Cal Davis scientists say they have convincing evidence that the chemical limits aren't enough. They don't even provide protection for prenatal infants. The scientists say this needs to be immediately addressed.

41. Medical Breakthrough Reverses Paralysis: Targeted Neurotechnology

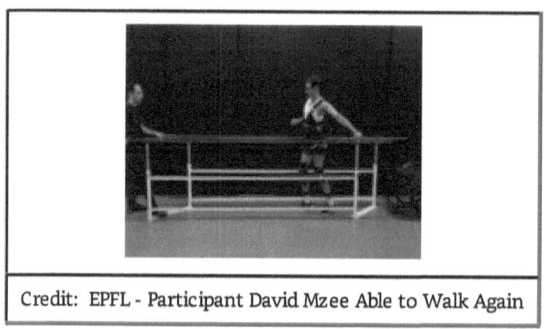

Credit: EPFL - Participant David Mzee Able to Walk Again

Significant Breakthrough for Spinal Cord Injuries

This is medicine at the cutting edge of innovation. Three patients with paraplegia were able to walk again when their spinal cords received electrical stimulation via a wireless implant. And after a few months of training the patients were able to control their previously paralyzed leg muscles without electrical stimulation. The three had significant spinal cord injuries.

Swiss Precision

The study was led by the Ecole Polytechnique Federale de

Lausanne and the Lausanne University Hospital in Switzerland. It establishes a new framework for improving recovery from spinal cord injuries.

Speedy and Effective Treatment
The patients, who had been paralyzed for years, regained voluntary control of their leg muscles within a week of treatment. The patients are able to walk on their own, with the aid of crutches or a walker. Through their extensive research, the scientists and physicians were able to mimic how the brain in real time naturally activates the spinal cord and triggers the growth of new nerve connections. The results were published in Nature and Nature Neuroscience.

42. Fitness Leads to Longer Life: Cleveland Clinic Landmark Research

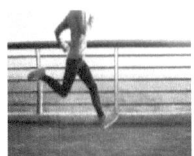

Source: Stock Photo

Cardiorespiratory Fitness is Key
Here's another great reason to even more enjoy your favorite exercise like running or biking. It's now proven to lead to a longer life. Researchers at the renowned Cleveland Clinic have found that cardiorespiratory fitness leads to a longer life. And they say there are no limits to the benefits of aerobic fitness.

Substantive, Long Term Research Results
This is a very substantive study. The research team retrospectively studied testing results on 122,007 patients who exercised on treadmills. The time frame is from January 1, 1991 thru December 31, 2014... more than 2 decades. The researchers meas-

ured all causes of mortality relating to fitness and exercise.

Aerobic Fitness Extends Life

The researchers say aerobic fitness is the key to a long life. And there is no limit on how much exercise is too much. According to the study's key author, cardiologist Wael Jaber, M.D., all of us should achieve high fitness levels. He added that the greatest benefits from top aerobic fitness come for people who are 70 plus and also for those with hypertension. Bottom-line: long term exercising has long term benefits. Have to love this great discovery on healthy living innovation and how important exercise is.

43. How Your Dog Understands Words: Emory University

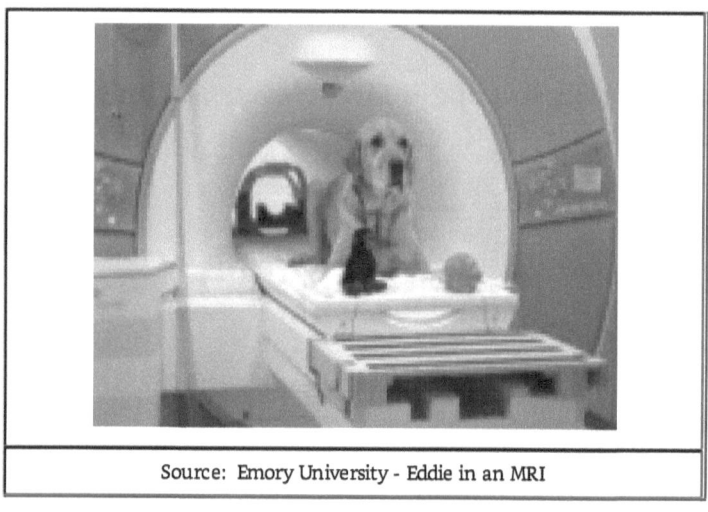

Source: Emory University - Eddie in an MRI

Fido's Brain

Scientists at Emory University have concluded that dogs have at the very minimum a basic neural representation of the meaning of words they've been taught. They differentiate between words they know and those they've never heard before.

Brain Imaging with Owners On Hand Giving Commands

This is one of the first studies using brain imaging to study how dogs process words associated with objects. We all know dogs learn to understand and obey verbal commands. But there is no substantive scientific evidence on how they do it.

Eddie and Friends

11 dogs joined Eddie, pictured above, in the Dog Project, along with their owners. The dogs were trained to voluntarily enter an MRI and remain motionless without any sedation while scanning occurred. Two objects, a stuffed animal and rubber toy, were used to monitor how the dogs associated the objects with words. The MRI's showed the auditory region of the brain showed greater activation on words the dogs never heard before, as though they were efforting to understand them.

Much Smarter than Just a Reflex Response

This is ongoing research and the beginning of the difficult process of mapping and understanding cognition in dogs' brains. But the scientists have already concluded that dogs have neural representation for words they've been taught, well beyond the Pavlovian response.

44. Smart Stickers that Monitor Heart: Purdue University Innovation

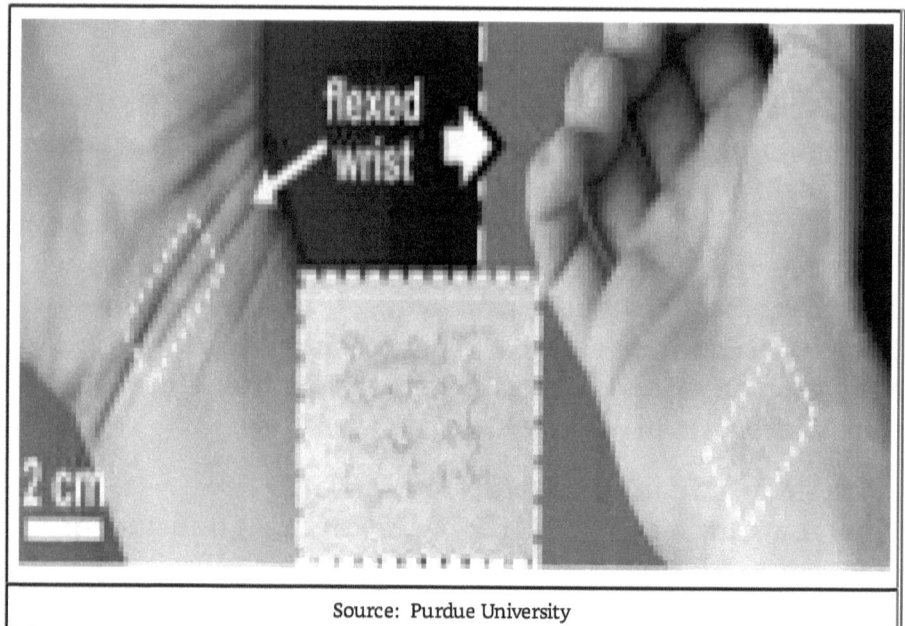

Source: Purdue University

Personal Health Monitoring that Costs 5 cents to Make

Scientists and engineers at Purdue have created a wearable, flexible, electronic sticker device that's easily attached to the skin. It monitors physical activity and can alert the user in real-time about possible health problems and risks. It can be used for patients, athletes and anyone who wants to monitor their health.

Personalized Medicine Made from Paper

It's made out of paper and costs only 5 cents to make. Not only is it wearable; it's nearly invisible. And it's biodegradable. This is the latest medical innovation that Purdue has contributed over the past 150 years. It is a history it's marking with its "Giant Leaps" celebration.

Available Very Soon

The smart stickers are composed of cellulose. They are biocompatible and breathable. They can also be implanted in the body for monitoring. They are expected to hit the market quickly as they are compatible with large-scale manufacturing.

45. Window into the Mind: Brain Cell Transplant Shows Brain Operating

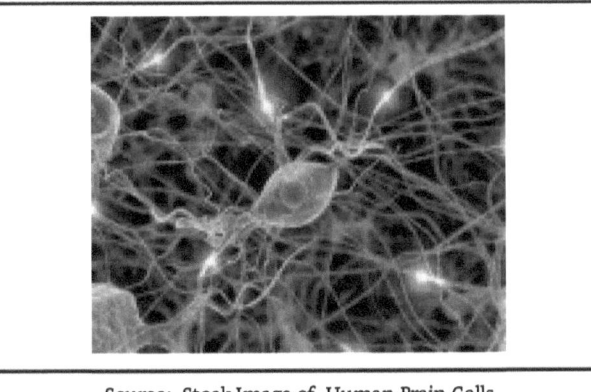

Source: Stock Image of Human Brain Cells

Breakthrough Neuroscience by Imperial College London

Scientists have created a window into the brain, which allows them to watch in real-time and with incredible details how human brain cells develop, connect and communicate with each other. The potential of their approach may result in better understanding of brain conditions like autism and provide eventual cures.

Volunteer Donators

Researchers from Imperial College London and the University of Cambridge transplanted human brain cells from volunteers into a mouse brain. It allowed them to study the way human brain cells interact in a natural environment.

Down Syndrome

The team used the technique to model Down Syndrome using brain cells donated by two individuals with the condition. They saw significant differences in the brain cells from those with Down Syndrome and those without it. They noted the cells are not as active as normal cells at a crucial stage of development.

Important to a Number of Brain Conditions

The medical research team says their approach can be used to study a range of brain conditions like dementia, Parkinson's, schizophrenia and autism. Their approach allows them to view in detail how cells communicate with each other. MRI's and PET scans aren't able to do that. The team is using a revolutionary microscopy technique - in vivo 2-photon microscopy - to see individual live brain cells and the connections between them.

46. Exercise Pumps Brain Power: Aerobics Improve Cognitive Performance

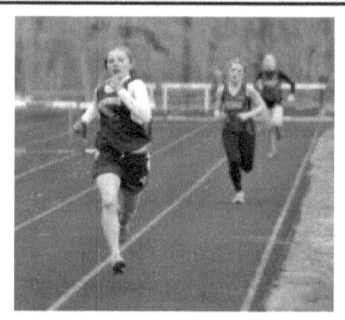

Source: Maryanne Kane's Photo of Katie Kane in Competition

Running to Prime Your Mind

Our brains are at their best when our bodies are in motion, like running, walking, biking rather than sedentary and sitting at a desk. A new study by German scientists just confirmed it. As a runner, I've always thought that I do my most deliberative thinking during a morning run. Now science confirms it. Wondered if as a jogger, biker, runner, walker and exerciser, you've had the same instincts? Do you do your best thinking in motion?

Active Motion Works

Scientists from Ludwig-Maximilian University in Germany took electroencephalogy brain readings on 24 participants when exercising and at rest. They found that exercise and upright posture improved visual working memory (that's the ability to maintain visual information to do ongoing tasks) significantly over passive and seated positions.

Counterintuitive From Centuries of Scholars Laboring at their Desks

This finding is fascinating and counterintuitive from our image of scholars working at their desks and also the fundamentals of cognitive science. Your mind primes in motion. The findings have been published in the British Journal of Psychology.

47. Infant's Brain Foreshadows the Adult's Emotional Control and Cognition

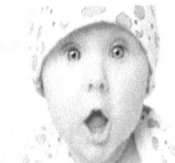

Source: Stock Image

UNC's Breakthrough Neuroscience Research

Medical researchers at University of North Carolina Health Care have made a remarkable series of discoveries. Using MRI's, they've shown that the brain circuits needed for successful emotional regulation in adults emerge in babies one to two years old. These brain circuits are the foundation of successful emotional development and IQ.

Predictors of Future Behavior and IQ

The growth rates of the emotion circuits in the brain during the child's second year "predict", according to the scientists, anxiety and emotional regulation at the age of four. It also predicts the child's IQ at the age of 4. Abnormal processing in the circuits is associated with depression, anxiety and schizophrenia in adults.

From the MRI's of Babies

The importance of these discoveries is the ability to foresee the individual's emotional control later in life but also their cognitive capabilities. It suggests to medical researchers new ways for early detection and intervention for children at risk for emotional problems and psychiatric disorders to reduce the risks and improve long-term behavioral outcomes. The results of this very substantive research involving 223 infants were published in Biological Psychiatry.

48. Type 2 Diabetes Reversed by Fasting

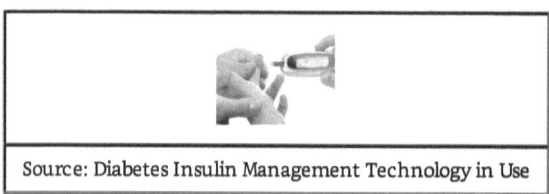

Source: Diabetes Insulin Management Technology in Use

Fasting Cuts Need for Insulin

Medical findings reported in the BMJ Case Report document that planned intermittent fasting may help to reverse Type 2 Diabetes. Three patients (in the care of doctors) who fasted were able to cut the need for insulin completely and quickly. With planned, intermittent fasting their blood glucose levels were back in control.

Diabetes is a Big Health Problem

1 in 10 people in the US and Canada have diabetes. It costs the US economy alone $245 billion per year. Drugs help patients control their diabetes but they don't stop the progression of the disease. Medical researchers have been searching for a cure for decades.

First, Preliminary but Impressive Results on Fasting

The findings are an informational study as only 3 patients, all men, are involved. The men have Type 2 Diabetes, high blood pressure and high cholesterol. Under their doctors' care, they tried fasting intermittently - essentially every other day. They've stayed with the regimen for ten months. One patient was off insulin in five days. The other two didn't need any insulin within a month. This is the first time that planned fasting was medically tried. The results are fascinating.

49. Vaccine Breakthrough: Universal, Cheaper, Stable Vaccines

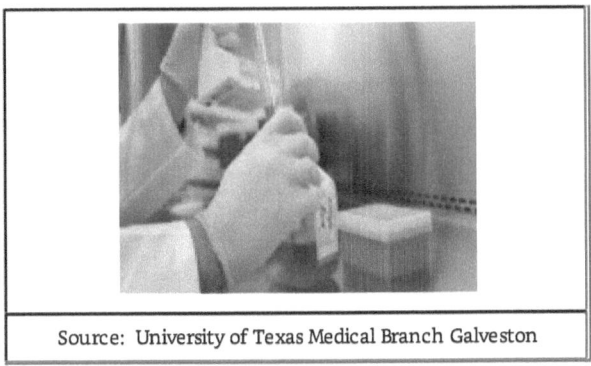

Source: University of Texas Medical Branch Galveston

DNA Vaccines that Could Impact World Health

Scientists at the University of Texas Medical Branch in Galveston have developed a universal vaccine platform. It cuts production and storage costs by 80%. It can be stockpiled at room temperature for years. And the new vaccines are as effective and safe as current vaccines.

DNA Based Immunizations

The breakthrough is that the scientists engineered the vaccines in DNA form. According to the scientists, testing proved a resounding success with the desired immunizations resulting.

Global Health Impact

The scientists' findings and their new vaccine methodology was published in EBioMedicine. This is of particular importance to hot, 3rd world countries where 80% of the vaccine cost comes from refrigeration.

50. How the Brain Computes: Rockefeller University Research

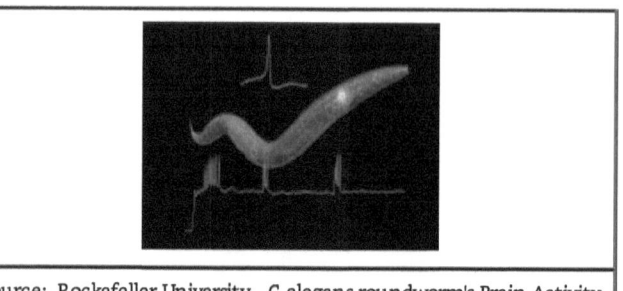

Source: Rockefeller University - C elegans roundworm's Brain Activity

In Tiny Worms, Spiking Neurons and Clues to Brain Function
The brain isn't a computer but it does compute. To process data the human brain uses a digital code. The cells produce bursts of electric current known as "action potentials". They are the 0's & 1's of the nervous system. The code is assumed to be vital also to animals.

Breakthrough Research on a Tiny Creature
Researchers at Rockefeller University have made an amazing discovery. They've had the world's first chance to observe "action potentials" in the brain cells of a tiny worm, the C elegans roundworm. It wasn't expected to be there. It's a first and experts say it is disrupting decades of dogma about the brain. And, it could help scientists understand fundamentals of brain computation.

Advancing Scientific Understanding of the Brain
The research team mapped all 302 neurons that make up the nervous system of C elegans and documented the unexpected "action potentials". They believe this will help to advance computational neuroscience and expand scientific understanding of the nervous system. The findings were published in the journal Cell.

51. Halt Aging: The Fountain of Youth in Fruits and Veggies

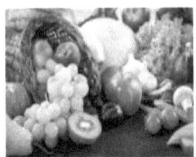

Source: Stock Image

Natural Substance Fisetin
University of Minnesota Medical School researchers have discovered a natural substance that intervenes and halts the aging process. The substance is called Fisetin and is found in many fruits and vegetables. It gives you all the more reason to eat lots of them.

Their Research Findings
The scientists treated aging mice with Fisetin. It has significant positive effects on health and lifespan. They published their study in EBioMedicine.

Healthspan Expansion
Their results suggest that the natural substance can extend the period of health called healthspan even late into life. But they do have a lot of questions to address such as proper dosage for individuals.

Science of Aging
As people age, they accumulate damaged cells. A younger person's immune system clears the cells. In older people, the cells aren't cleared as effectively. The accumulation results in deteriorating tissue and aging. The scientists found Fisetin positively intervened in the process. They call it a senotherapeutic that extends health and lifespan.

52. Implantable Health Trackers: 24/7 Medical Biomarker Monitoring

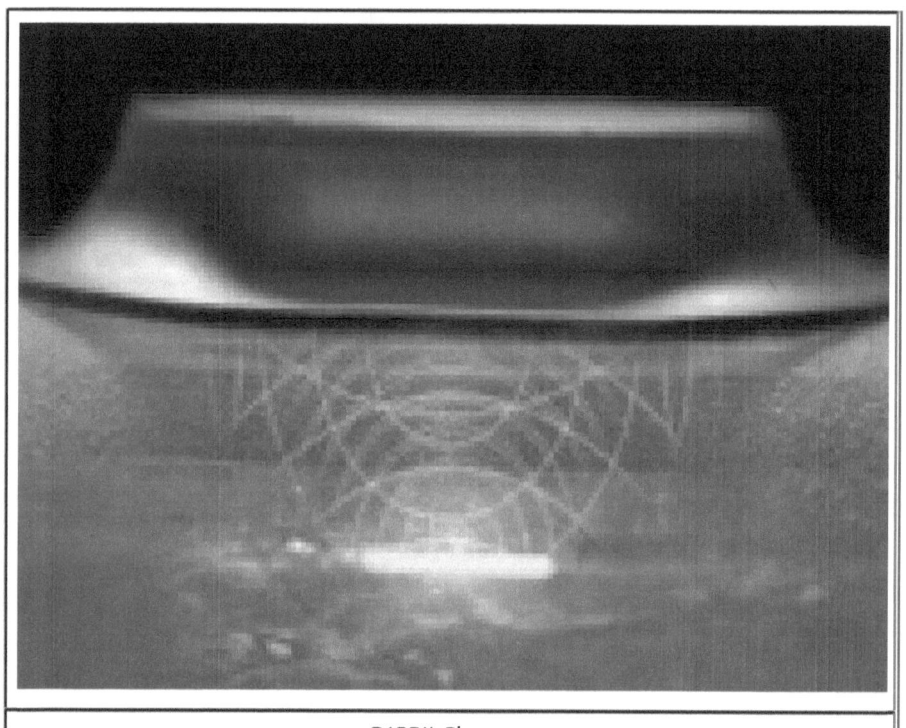

DARPA's Biosensor

Connects to Devices Like Smartphones

You know when you don't feel well. But this advanced research would take monitoring your health to a whole new level. Implantable health trackers are futuristic technology being developed right now for delivery ASAP. It's called tissue-integrated biosensor technology and it's being developed by the US Army Research Office and DARPA, the US Defense Department's Advanced Research Projects Agency.

Biosensors

The biosensors are tiny, soft, hydrogel-based sensors implanted under the skin. The purpose is to use them to measure biomarkers related to oxygen, lactate, urea, glucose and ion levels. The sensors can stay in the human body for up to 2 years. They can read out information to connected devices such as smartphones.

General Public Use
Every project that DARPA undertakes is aimed at providing the US military with overwhelming technological advantages against adversaries. Like many other DARPA innovation discoveries such as GPS, the internet, flying cars and cloud computing, there's a tremendous benefit to the public. This same technology could one day help individuals manage difficult chronic diseases that need constant monitoring like diabetes.

53. Heart Monitor Taped on Skin: Organic Sensor & Organic Solar Cell

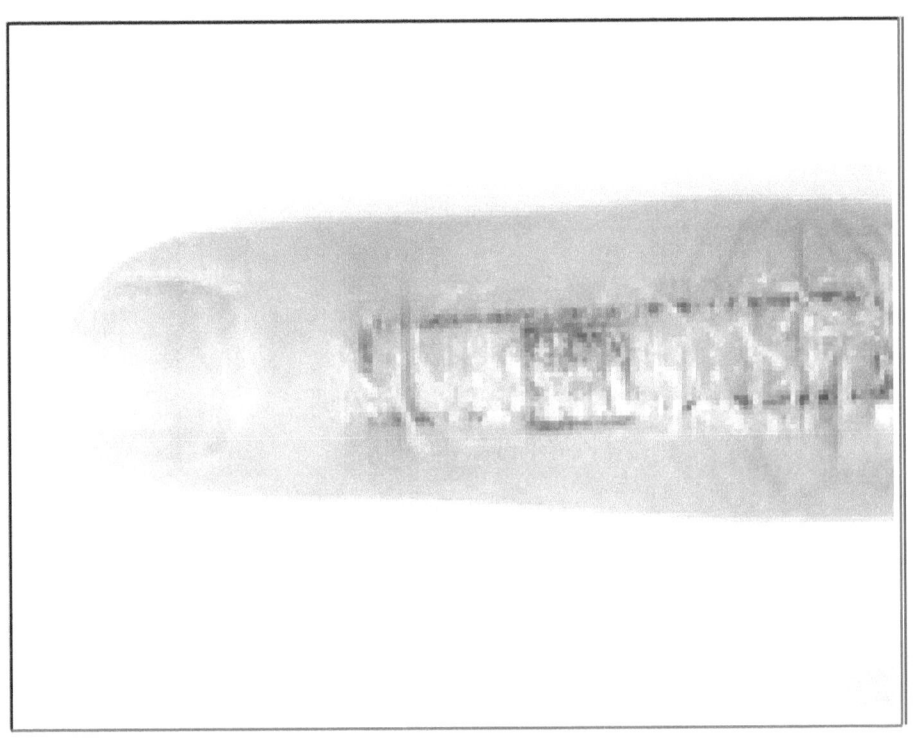

Source: RIKEN Center

Very Flexible, Taped Heart Monitor on Your Finger
Scientists have developed an organic sensor powered by sunlight that performs as a self-powered heart monitor. The scientists put a sensor device, an organic, electrochemical transistor, into a flexible organic solar cell. The device successfully measures the heartbeats of humans under bright light conditions.

New Generation of Self-Medical Monitoring
This monitor, developed by scientists at the RIKEN Center for Emergent Matter Science and the University of Tokyo, is easy to use and ultra flexible with a solar powered sensor. It can also be used to monitor brain function. The development was reported in the journal Nature. It's being hailed as the next generation of self-medical monitoring. Such self-powered devices placed on the skin have great potential for medical monitoring applications.

54. Ending Malaria By Gene Mutation

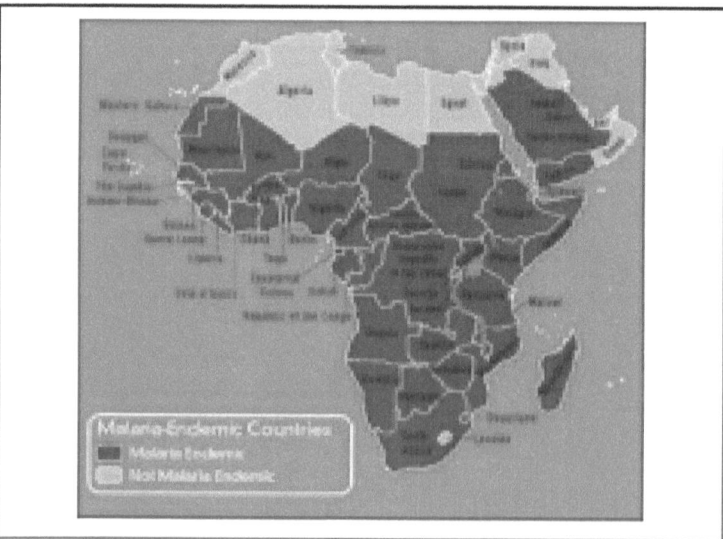

Source: Africa's Malaria-Endemic Countries

DNA Editing

Malaria is among the world's worst scourges. In Africa in 2016, 194 million people were infected by malaria and nearly half a million died from it. The deadly disease is caused by a parasite and transmitted by mosquito bites.

Imperial College London Biologists

A team of biologists at Imperial College London may have the weapon to end the scourge. They've successfully gene-edited mosquitos to self-destruct. They've targeted a patch of DNA that never varies. By gene editing the female mosquitos into infertility, the population becomes extinct within 5 to 11 generations.

Potential: Malaria Eliminated within 2 Decades

If this gene editing is as successful as lab tests have been, the scientists believe malaria could be eliminated within 2 decades. Computer models indicate that in the wild mosquito populations could be made extinct by the technique within 4 years.

55. Membrane Controls Blood Pressure: Promise of Better Treatments

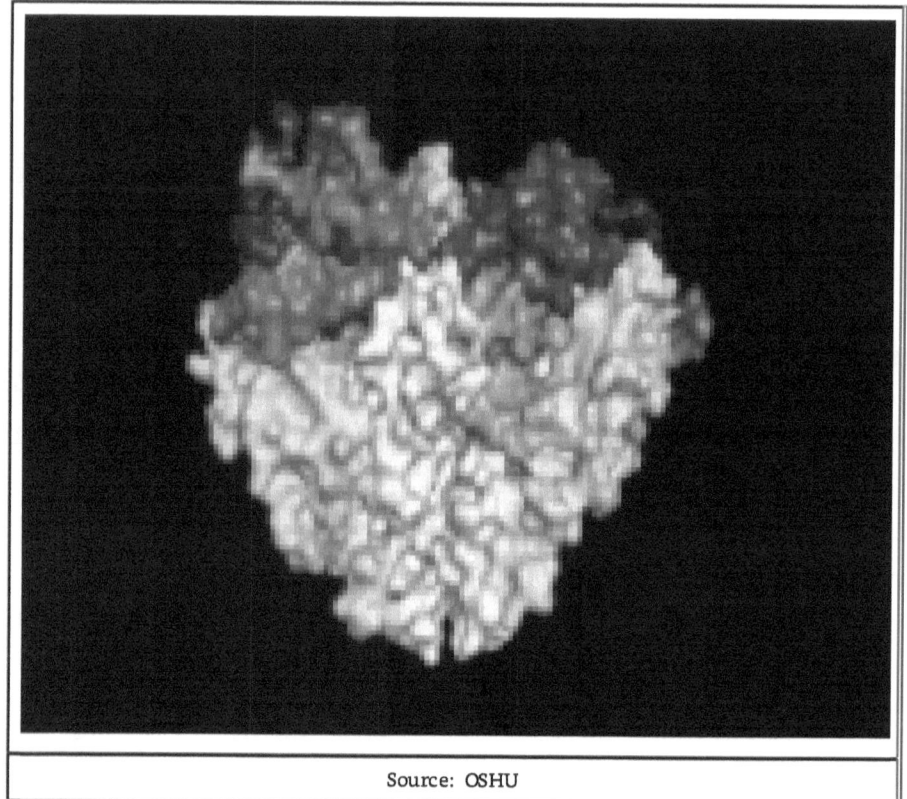

Source: OSHU

Breakthrough Research by Oregon Health and Science University

New research by scientists at Oregon Health & Science University in Portland reveals the 3-dimensional structure of a membrane that controls blood pressure. The membrane is called the human epithelial sodium channel. It has never been as precisely isolated and detailed as that done by the OHSU researchers.

Membrane Is Critical to Human Health

Using a cyro-electron microscope, the researchers generated a 3D model of the channel. Besides being critical to controlling blood pressure, it's also impactful on other functions in the body. The channel enables sodium ions to be absorbed into tissue through-out the body including the kidney. As such, it's critical to human health by regulating sodium balance, blood volume and blood pressure.

Great Potential for New Therapies

This discovery is expected to lead to new and better blood pressure treatments. Researchers also believe it will enable targeted, customized medication for heart failure, nephrotic syndrome as well as severe hypertension. The breakthrough research was published in the journal eLife.

56. Can Organ Transplants Cause Cancer? Very Rare but Yes

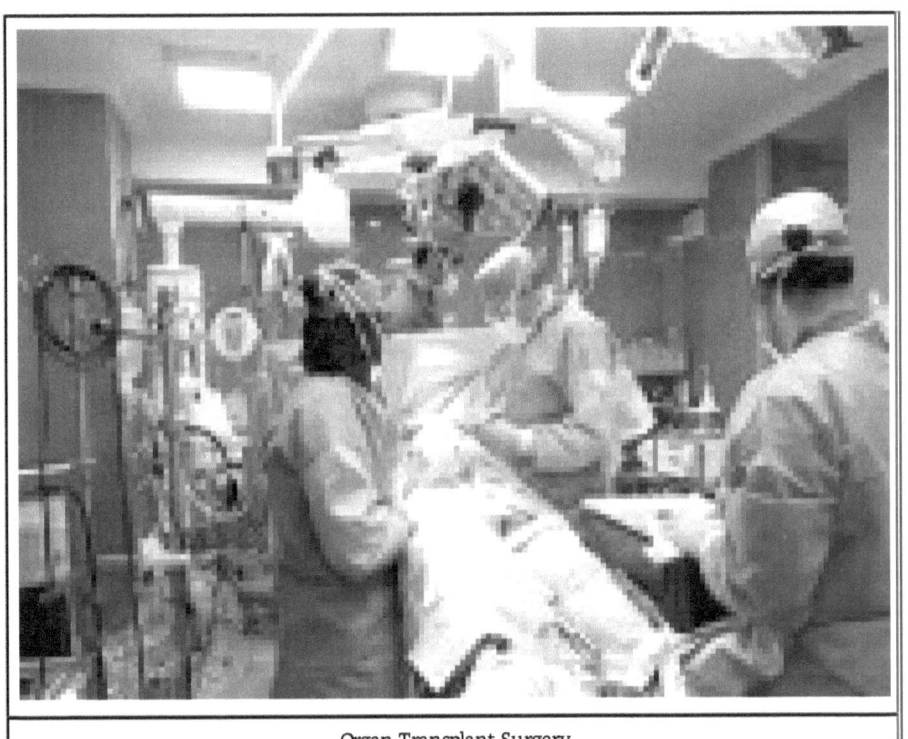

Organ Transplant Surgery

European Case

It's well known that organ transplants can pass on infectious diseases from the donor to the recipient in rare cases. New scientific research shows that passing cancer from a donor to a transplant recipient is extraordinarily rare but can happen. In fact, a donor's undetectable cancer cells caused 4 transplant recipients, including a man, to develop breast cancer. 3 of them died. This case emerged in Europe and was published in the scientific journal Transplant.

Donor History of No Detectable Cancer
The 53 yr old donor died of a stroke and had no detectable signs of cancer. But doctors traced back the DNA in the cancer cells found in the 4 recipients. The DNA matched that of the donor. Scientists say the chance of something like this happening is 1 to 5 in 10,000 cases. But, it's important research findings and something to be aware of. The incidences are extraordinary rare but possible.

57. Smart Phone Ultrasounds: Could Lower Scan Cost to $100

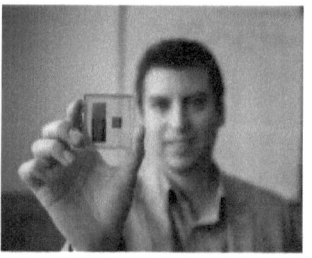

Photo: University of BC Lead Researcher Carlos Gerardo with new the transducer

Potential Use for 24/7 Self-Monitoring by Smart Phone
Engineers at the University of British Columbia have developed a new ultrasound transducer or probe. It could lower the cost of an ultrasound scan to $100. This is patent-pending breakthrough

tech. It's portable, wearable and can be powered by your smart phone. It's no bigger than a band-aide. The researchers say the potential is endless and could provide 24/7 monitoring of your arteries and veins to warn of the danger of heart attack or stroke.

How Did They Do It?

To simplify, they replaced piezoelectric crystals used to create images and deliver sonograms in conventional scanners with tiny vibrating drums of polymer resin. The cost saving is dramatic and the image quality is as good as or better than conventional systems according to published reports. The UBC transducer needs only 10 volts to operate and can be powered by a smart phone.

Next Steps

Clinical tests need to be done. But there's another fascinating aspect to this tech. Researchers say it has the potential to be further miniaturized and built into flexible material that could wrap around the body for easier scanning and more detailed images, including 24/7 monitoring of arteries and veins.

58. Probiotics Unequal Benefits

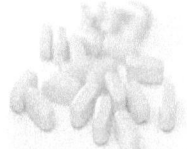

Source: Stock Image of Probiotics

Israeli Study Finds Unequal Benefits

Many people take probiotics through food and supplements to boost their digestive health. Israeli scientists at the Weizmann Institute of Science have released a study that shows the so-called "good bacteria" benefits some people more than others. And in fact it sometimes can do more harm than good.

Customized Probiotics

The scientists suggest a new approach to the use of probiotics. Their conclusion is that probiotics should not be given out as a "1 size fits all supplement". Instead they should be individualized based on the microbes present in the person's stomach to maximize beneficial results. They also discovered that probiotics can have a potentially harmful effect if given after antibiotics. Their study was published in the journal Cell.

59. Gene Editing MS: Successful Treatment on Dogs

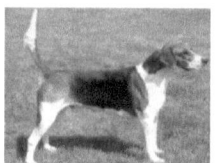

Source: Stock Image

London and Dallas Research Team
For the first time, there is real hope for a potential cure for Muscular Dystrophy. A team of scientists from the Royal Veterinary College in London and UT Southwestern Medical College in Dallas used gene therapy on dogs with the disease. They repaired a gene mutation that triggers the fatal condition.

Editing DNA
This is an important step in the process to edit DNA in people with the fatal disease. 20,000 children, mostly boys, are diagnosed with it every year. Muscular Dystrophy is caused by a gene mutation that stops production of dystrophin, a protein that's essential to healthy muscle function. Without the protein muscles dramatically deteriorate.

More Research
The research was published in the journal Science. The scientists successfully used gene editing in four dogs with the disease. The procedure restored the production of dystrophin in the animals.

Experts say much more research will be required before they can utilize it on humans.

60. First Human X-Rays in Living Color

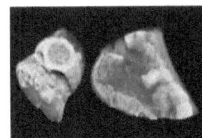

Source: MARS Bioimaging

Straight From MARS and Absolutely Amazing
New Zealand-based MARS Bioimaging has created the world's first color X-rays of the human body. The company is an award winning manufacturer of small bore spectral CT scanners. The scans are 3D and used for pre-clinical medical research.

In Depth, In Color
The CT scanners produce color images where different materials can be separated. In the above photo, soft tissue, fat, bone and the metal of a watch are all identified and differentiated. The company explains this is photon counting technology, originally created as part of MARS founder's work at CERN, the European Organization for Nuclear Research.

Medical Research Benefits
The benefit for researchers is the wealth of precise chemical data on objects in the scanner. The careful, multilayers of tissue scans, the company says, enable new precision in medical research. To do this, MARS has placed sensors inside computed tomography (CT) scanners. By matching the scans with how different chemical compounds interact with X-ray light, they're able to pinpoint what chemical compounds are present in living tissue. You might say it's bloody amazing.

61. Sleep Essential For Learning

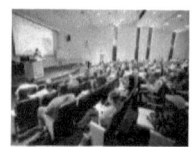

Source: Stock Photo

All Nighters Don't Work

Students should make sleep an educational priority. A good night's sleep is essential for human memory. Neuroscientists are just starting to understand why. All nighters don't work for exams. In fact, they're the worst thing you can do.

UK Sleep Research

Scientists at the Royal Holloway University in the United Kingdom have documented that sleep is essential to embedding knowledge in the brain. Sleep affects memory, especially the recall needed to learn language.

To Sleep or Not to Sleep

The researchers documented two groups of students learning new vocabulary words. The group that got a good night's sleep far outperformed the group that studied all night. The bottom line: prolonged sleep is actually good for kids and adults. It's critical for brain function and healthy body rhythms. And, for students, it's a priority for better test performance and grades.

62. Reversing Paralysis: New Brain Implant Size of Matchstick

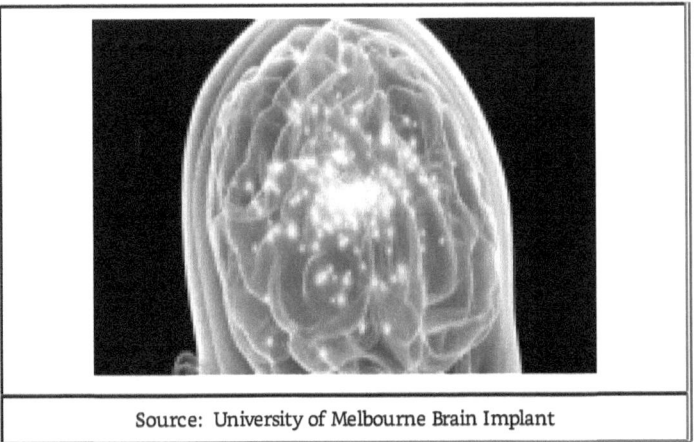

Source: University of Melbourne Brain Implant

In Australia, University of Melbourne bioengineers have developed a brain implant the size of a matchstick, that may help people paralyzed walk again. It's been successfully tested on sheep.

Stentrode
The implant is called Stentrode. It circumvents the spinal cord and enables movement driven by the person's thoughts. It's a tiny device containing electrodes.

DARPA and Australian Government Research Funding
The US Defense Department's Advanced Research Projects Agency DARPA and the Government of Australia have funded the research. The research team hopes to test the Stentrode on five volunteers.

Wireless Thoughts
The system relays thoughts wirelessly to an external robotic device such as an exoskeleton or prosthetic limb. The Stentrode enables patient-directed, brain control over movement and locomotion.

Human Augmentation
The Stentrode device is part of the growing field of robotics for human augmentation. By 2025, this sector is forecast to be a $2 trillion industry. 50 million people around the world have im-

paired mobility and could greatly benefit.

63. Gut Check by e-Pill: Electronic Capsule, Diagnostic and Dietary Tech

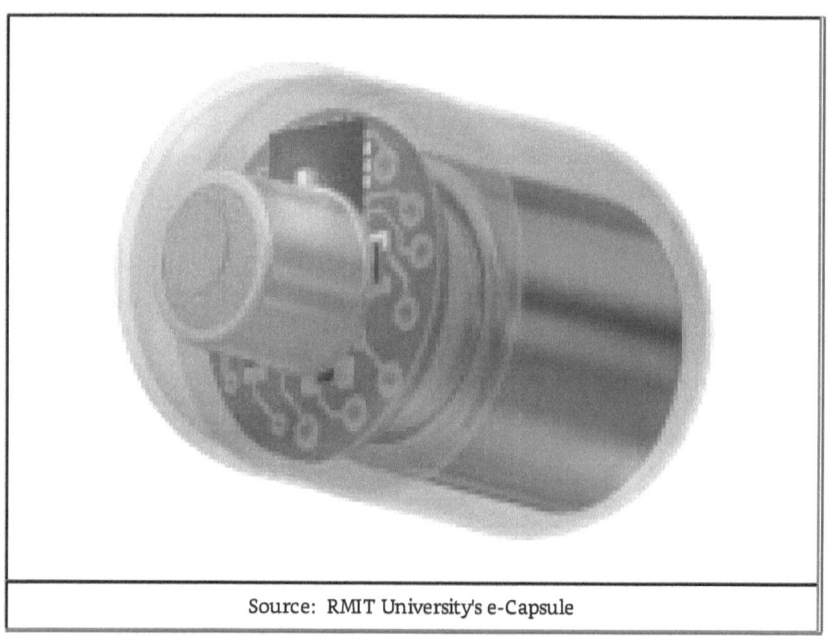

Source: RMIT University's e-Capsule

New e-Pill
In Australia, RMIT University scientists have developed an ingestible electronic capsule. It provides a potentially powerful diagnostic technique and unique information on the effects of diet and medical supplements. The pill is loaded with highly advanced sensors that monitor and measure.

Individualized, Precision Diets
The e-capsule could help to develop individualized, precision diets. It precisely monitors what's present in the stomach and intestinal track, including oxygen, CO_2, hydrogen and microbes. According to the RMIT scientists, it safely and accurately measures the effects of diet - what's working and what isn't. The e-pill also has the potential of working as a powerful diagnostic tool.

24/7 Information On Cell Phone

The e-capsule monitors 24/7. It sends the data real-time to a monitor that displays on a cell phone. Every five minutes it also displays the information on a hand-held monitor. This break-through device could have significant value for personalized medicine including individualized drug therapies.

64. Converting Stem Cells to Nerve Cells: Reversing Paralysis

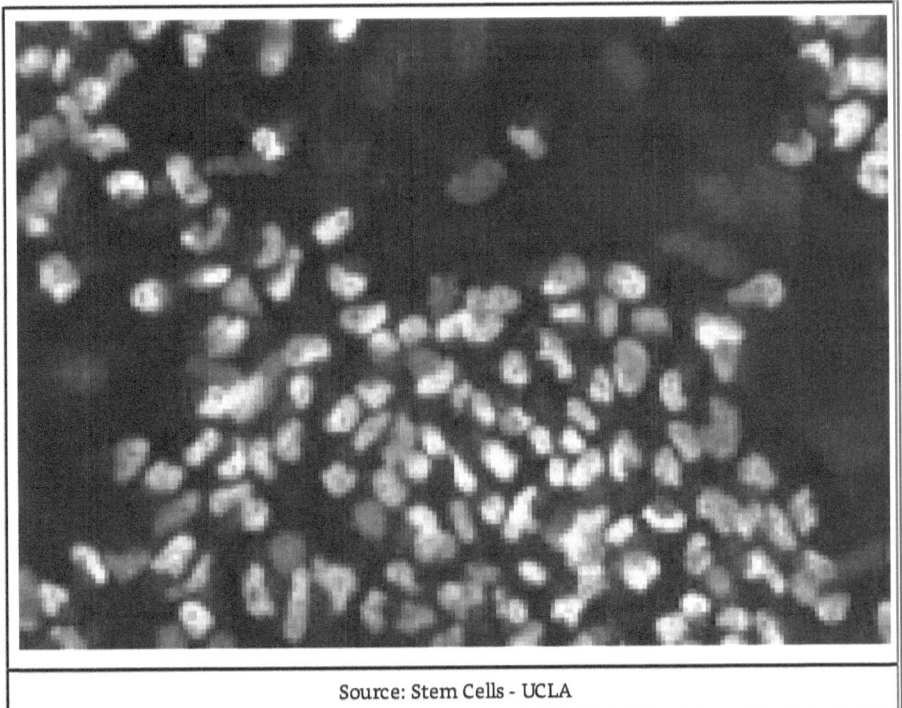

Source: Stem Cells - UCLA

Cellular Pathways

Researchers at UCLA have turned human stem cells into sensory interneurons. These are the cells that give us a sense of touch. This could be a step toward stem-cell based therapies to restore feeling in people who are paralyzed and have lost sensation in parts of their body.

Neurons

Sensory interneurons are a type of neuron in the spinal cord. They relay information from throughout the body to the central nervous system, which enables a sense of touch. Creating nerve cells from stem cells is a first. The researchers also did so while maintaining the genetic code of the person they originated from. That's important because the scientists say it eliminates immune suppression.

Ongoing Research with Significant Potential

Lead researcher Asso. Prof. Samantha Butler noted that you need to be able to feel and sense your body in space in order to walk. Feeling and walking go hand-in-hand. This breakthrough research could eventually lead to cell-based treatments for paralysis.

65. Medical Breakthrough with Virtual Reality

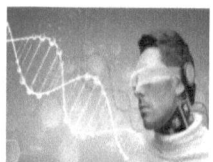

Source: EPFL

Swiss Medical Innovation

Scientists at Switzerland's Ecole Polytechnique Federale de Lausanne (EPFL) combined virtual reality with artificial tactile sensation to help two amputees feel their prosthetic hand as part of their body. They also demonstrated that the phantom limb actually grows into the prosthetic hand.

Mind-Body-VR Connections

The basis of this breakthrough approach is how the brain identifies what belongs to its own body. Their breakthrough was combining two senses - sight and touch. According to the lead scientist Giulio Rognini of EPFL: "We showed exactly how vision and touch can be combined to trick the amputee's brain into feeling what it sees" thru VR.

Portable Therapy

This process is portable and could be turned into therapy to help patients embody their prosthetic limbs permanently. It's a case of VR providing life enhancing feeling and experience.

66. Lab on a Chip: Medical Tests Possible on Coin Sized Chip

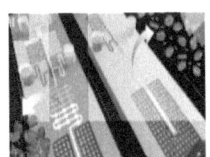

Source: University of Buffalo

University of Buffalo Success

Researchers at the University of Buffalo have done what many others have tried without success. They're created medical tests on a chip the size of a coin. They've demonstrated how their chip accurately determines the eight blood types based on the time it takes each to flow thru the chip.

Medical Tech Breakthrough

This is a breakthrough. The obstacle has been finding a reliable and efficient way to mix and move blood and other fluids thru a chip's tiny pumps and valves. The UB team have done it. They fabricated a chip that uses two different types of forces - capillary & vacuum driven - to move the fluids in micro and nanosized channels. This advance solves a difficult problem that has been an obstacle to labs on a chip.

Big Vision for Medical Labs on Chips

The expectations for the use of labs on chips are big, including in the developing world, on battlefields and in our homes. Imagine, you put a pinprick of your blood on the chip to see if you have strep throat or the flu. This is personalized medicine and medical technology at the cutting edge.

University of Buffalo Advancement

The new chip requires no sensors or external power source. It advances what the medical world is looking for: inexpensive and disposable labs on chips that are fast, reliable, inexpensive and self-administered.

67. Penn's Mind Stimulator: Gentle Electric Pulse Boosts Memory

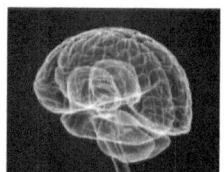

Source: Stock Image

University of Pennsylvania Innovation

Scientists at the University of Pennsylvania have demonstrated that gentle, imperceptible electric impulses passing through the brain improve memory and information retention.

15% Improvement

In fact, the electric pulses increase memory and information retention up to 15%. The electrical stimulation is precisely timed and targeted to the left side of the brain in the left lateral temporal cortex.

Real-Time

The Penn team developed a system to monitor the brain's activity real-time and trigger stimulation based on the activity. The electrical pulses are unfelt and at a safe level.

Exciting, Personalized Machine Learning Models

Twenty five neurosurgical patients being treated for epilepsy participated in the study at clinical sites around the US. The scientists developed patient-specific, personalized machine learning models. They programmed the stimulator to deliver pulses only when memory was predicted to fail. That gives the technology the best chance to restore memory.

Tremendous Potential

This is early stage research with very promising results. The potential application and importance of this technology for patients with memory loss from age, disease, stroke and trauma are of great interest.

www.ingramcontent.com/pod-product-compliance
Lightning Source LLC
Chambersburg PA
CBHW032103280526
45784CB00013B/3009